Copernicus Books

Sparking Curiosity and Explaining the World

Drawing inspiration from their Renaissance namesake, Copernicus books revolve around scientific curiosity and discovery. Authored by experts from around the world, our books strive to break down barriers and make scientific knowledge more accessible to the public, tackling modern concepts and technologies in a nontechnical and engaging way. Copernicus books are always written with the lay reader in mind, offering introductory forays into different fields to show how the world of science is transforming our daily lives. From astronomy to medicine, business to biology, you will find herein an enriching collection of literature that answers your questions and inspires you to ask even more.

Petros Perros

Seeking Thyroid Truths

A Guide for the Curious

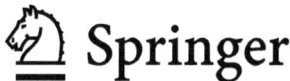 Springer

Petros Perros
Institute of Translational and Clinical Research
Newcastle University
Newcastle upon Tyne, UK

Copernicus Books
ISSN 2731-8982   ISSN 2731-8990   (electronic)
Sparking Curiosity and Explaining the World
ISBN 978-3-031-58286-8   ISBN 978-3-031-58287-5   (eBook)
https://doi.org/10.1007/978-3-031-58287-5

Illustrations by Giorgos Perros

This Springer imprint is published by the registered company Springer Nature Switzerland AG
The registered company address is: Gewerbestrasse 11, 6330 Cham, Switzerland

If disposing of this product, please recycle the paper.

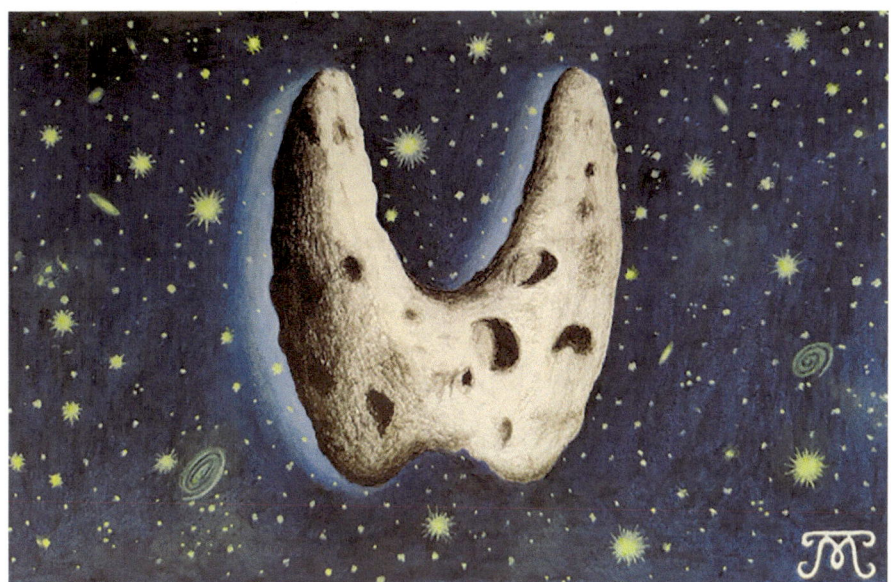

What could space possibly have to do with the thyroid? NASA astronauts on the Space Shuttle programme had numerous tests before and after flights. Thyroid blood tests showed some abnormalities after flights in the early expeditions. This was due to iodine being used to purify water. In later Space Shuttle flights, measures were taken to remove iodine from drinking water [1]

To Shirin, Tash, Ali and Adam

Prologue

'The intention of this book is to provide the means by which good quality information about the thyroid gland and its diseases can be found, accessed, weighed and judged'

Who Is This Book for and What Is It About?

This book is for patients with thyroid diseases and anyone interested in the thyroid, including carers of thyroid patients, members of the lay public, medical students and healthcare workers (nurses, pharmacists, trainees in endocrinology, family doctors) who deal with patients. The focus in on the thyroid, but the concepts apply to any field of medicine if the reader is interested in exploring and understanding the evidence, while thyroid themes are used as examples.

There are numerous questions relating to the thyroid that the best experts are unable to answer with certainty, yet people with thyroid problems have to make judgements that affect their health. Doctors for a variety of reasons often do not deliver the amount and depth of information needed by those who suffer from thyroid diseases. Inevitably such information is sought elsewhere, usually the internet. The end result is frequently confusing, disappointing and sometimes perilous. This book will not offer opinions about why you may be having problems with your thyroid, nor will it encourage you to spend your money on remedies of questionable value. The intention is to provide the means by which good quality information about the thyroid gland and its diseases can be found, accessed, weighed and judged. It will hopefully enable you to assess the quality of the information and make good decisions about health. It is a guide that can lead you to the original sources of up-to-date knowledge and help you answer your questions. To do so, you will need to navigate treacherous waters and dodge misinformation, bias, conspiracy theories and a multitude of opinions often based on other people's opinions. *Seeking Thyroid Truths* is a companion for such a journey. The reader can refer to it time and again when faced with specific questions about the thyroid to help with the search. The book also contains anecdotes and explanatory examples and can be read like a story. Besides practical advice about finding and assessing medical evidence, I offer my own opinions in the last chapter, on a specific topic of great importance (in my opinion). It would be foolish to claim impartiality though care was taken to minimise it.

Success in finding truth is not guaranteed, in fact that would be a highly unrealistic expectation, but an Odyssean journey may be rendered less Herculean.

Acknowledgements

My wife Shirin deserves my endless gratitude for her encouragement and infinite tolerance. I am thankful to family, friends, colleagues and patients for their feedback and advice: Dr. Denise Adams, Roger Ashworth, Dr. Arie Berghout, Professor David S Cooper, Kate Farnell, Joan Grant, Professor Laszlo Hegedüs, Janis Hickey, Professor Marian Ludgate, Dr. Ujjal Mallick, Giannis Mandaltsis, Professor Pat Kendall-Taylor, Margaret McGregor, Cheryl McMullen, Elspeth Ross, Giorgos Perros, Dr. Tash Perros, Ali Perros, Dr. Adam Perros, Dr. Alan Poots, Julia Priestley, Anna Reavel, Wendy Scott and Maggie Waugh. George Priestley kindly provided the photograph of the house where Bernard Courtoise (discoverer of iodine) was born. Golis Ligas captured a magnificent Aegean sunset from Athos in the back cover. I am particularly grateful to my brother Giorgos Perros who, inspired by thyroid themes, created the artwork.

Introduction

'Those who argue against empowering people without a PhD in health sciences, underestimate their ability.'

A Star Patient

I remember my first day as a consultant like it was yesterday, from the moment I woke up, to entering the office where my predecessor's presence still lingered, to my first outpatient clinic on the same afternoon, to getting home in the evening eager to tell my family about my new job. It was a great day and the variety of endocrine cases that crossed the threshold of my consulting room was beyond my expectations.

My encounter with my star patient, a man called Vero, happened a few weeks later. His family doctor rang me during my morning ward round. She sounded very excited and wanted to forewarn me that a referral was on its way about the most amazing case of 'myxoedema' that she had ever seen and would I like him to get started on levothyroxine immediately? I offered to see Vero the same afternoon and 3 h later there he was. He came from Serbia and had recently travelled to the UK to join his cousin's family. He was only 52 but looked much older. He shuffled into my consulting room accompanied by his cousin who also acted as a translator. He slowly lowered himself into the chair and stayed motionless, apathetic, almost lifeless. His skin was like parchment and slightly yellow, the tissues around his eyes puffy, his hands were freezing cold, his pulse slow and his feet swollen. When prompted to answer my questions, it became obvious that he was hard of hearing, his voice was gruff, his speech slow, his tongue too big for his mouth and he had a 'goitre' (enlarged thyroid gland). 'Myxoedema' is a medical term that means severe thyroid underactivity. And Vero indeed had myxoedema at its most extreme. The lab tests were as expected 'off the scale' and the reports had stars all over highlighting that the 'TSH was greater than 100 mU/L' and the 'free T4 less than 1 pmol/L'.

Vero had lived all his life in a remote village in the mountainous region between Serbia and Bulgaria. Access to healthcare was difficult and it seemed that during his teenage years he had started to develop the symptoms that he now presented with. You may be surprised to know (as was his family doctor) that I did not treat Vero with thyroid hormones. There were three clues that made me doubt that this was straightforward hypothyroidism (thyroid underactivity), of the type that we usually see in the developed world ('Hashimoto's thyroiditis' or 'autoimmune hypothyroidism'): (a) he was a man (in the UK more than 90% of people with hypothyroidism are female), (b) he came from a mountainous area, (c) he had a goitre. These suggested that the underlying problem was not destruction of his thyroid gland due to Hashimoto's thyroiditis, but lack of the raw material (iodine) that the thyroid needs for making thyroid hormones. Additional tests confirmed that he was severely iodine deficient. Being somewhat concerned that he may not be able to take iodine supplements by mouth consistently, I leaned on my colleagues in pharmacy who were very kind to respond to my highly unusual request for an injection of iodinated oil, which repletes the body of iodine for over a year. Vero walked into my consulting room a new man a few months later. He was animated, talkative and looked the picture of health. He never came back despite multiple invitations for clinic appointments. I took that to be a good sign of someone who had recovered completely and had no need to see an endocrinologist and hopefully adhering to the dietary advice that he was given. I was not destined ever to encounter another case of myxoedema as striking as this for the rest of my career as an endocrinologist.

As recently as the late nineteenth century, doctors would not have been able to help patients like Vero. His story is an example of how science expands our knowledge, which when applied can change people's destiny for the better. What drives science is our desire to unravel truth. This yearning has a long history and is one of the defining characteristics of our species.

Seeking Truths

Seeking truths implies knowledge of what truth is. This has preoccupied some of the best minds in the history of mankind, often driving them to insanity. I have avoided entering that philosophical battleground and have assumed that there is a common understanding of what we consider true in our daily lives. Where and how to look for it is a condition for reaching the evidence, but then you have to decide whether your bounty is truthful, and that is the centre of attention in this book.

Two and a half thousand years ago, Aristotle and Plato wrestled with ideas about truth in their own way, and this struggle was captured by a great artist on one of the walls of the Vatican. My first encounter with that fresco in real life planted the seeds for writing this book.

Aristotle and Plato

My first visit to the Vatican Museum came late in life. Previous experiences of places like the British Museum, the Louvre and the Uffizi Gallery, were marked by an intense sense of awe and emotional fatigue triggered by the abundance and magnificence of what was displayed.

'Florence syndrome' is known to afflict some people who come face to face with objects of exceptional beauty and causes a collection of physical and mental symptoms [2]. Whether I suffered from it I am not sure. But the feeling of personal worthlessness in comparison to the creators of such works was overwhelming, as I staggered out of the Uffizi Gallery onto the north bank of the Arno on a scorching August afternoon in 2006.

When it came to the Vatican Museum, I was better prepared. I decided I would concentrate on one room (the Sistine Chapel) and specifically the paintings on the ceiling and the altar wall by the great Michelangelo Buonarroti.

Reaching the Sistine Chapel entails walking through long corridors full of opulent Renaissance art, which invites the visitor's attention and is highly seductive. But I remained composed and I surprised even myself for resisting the distractions beckoning from all directions.

I was nearly at the entrance of the Sistine Chapel, full of anticipation and excitement, when my defences were breached by the sight of Raphael's 'The School of Athens'.

Aristotle the empiricist points down to earth, while Plato the visionary draws attention to the skies. Both men were in search of knowledge and truth, but they differed in their opinions of how to reach them (Fig. 1). I was mesmerised by this gigantic and magnificent fresco. It took my breath away and delayed my entry into the Sistine Chapel by some 30 min of jaw-dropped staring.

Choosing the word 'truth' as part of the title of this book was not a hasty nor an easy decision. It carries a heavy weight and implies a promise for unveiling truth, which is burdensome. So, writing about the truth in relation to the thyroid turned out to be a bigger challenge than I thought.

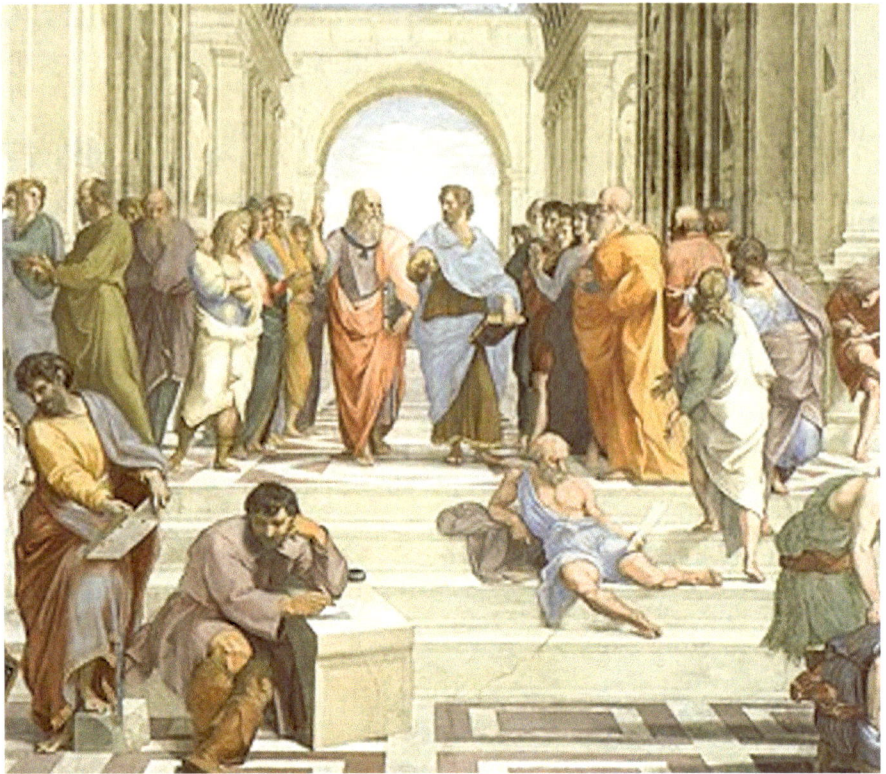

Fig. 1 The School of Athens by Raphael [3]

In medicine and in science, truth is pursued through 'empirical' knowledge, which tallies with Aristotle's teachings. That is, observation, experimentation, collection of facts and analysis, from where conclusions are drawn and 'hypotheses' (assumptions or theories) are constructed. Such hypotheses have to be testable, otherwise they are meaningless. A hypothesis that thyroid cancer is caused by genetic 'mutations' (or faults) can be explored by comparing genes from thyroid cancer cells with non-cancerous tissue. To propose that 'hypothyroidism is blue' is impossible to test scientifically although it may carry some literary value.

Truth occasionally reveals itself in a manner that defies doubt. There are instances when it is anticipated and expected like the last piece in a jigsaw puzzle. When it finally arrives, it is accepted with little hesitation because it is a perfect fit. In the late 1980s, a race was well on its way to find the gene for the 'TSH receptor'. The TSH receptor is a protein that sits on the surface of thyroid cells onto which TSH (thyroid-stimulating hormone, made in the pituitary, which is another gland) docks in and switches on many functions of thyroid cells.

Several laboratories all over the world dedicated financial resources, time, effort and brain power to find the TSH receptor gene. Such great interest was justified not only because of the central importance of the TSH receptor in how thyroid cells work, but also because it could bring better understanding of thyroid diseases and open up opportunities for new treatments. The TSH receptor gene was eventually found and a truth emerged about its precise location and the sequence of the DNA building blocks that made up the gene. It was then possible to synthesise it, transplant it in bacteria, yeasts or non-thyroid human cells and it functioned and behaved as predicted. Cracking the TSH receptor gene has expanded our understanding and new treatments are currently in development as a result.

Other truths are much more elusive. The documentation that some patients with hypothyroidism continue to experience symptoms despite receiving treatment is one such example. Numerous studies have been performed over the past 30 years and we understand this phenomenon a little better now, but it largely remains unsolved, and it is already evident that it will not be as simple as a missing piece in a puzzle.

In health sciences, the other face of truth is the living experiences of people afflicted with illness. Knowledge that comes from scientific studies and living experiences of patients are two separate ways to the truth. They both have their own limitations, but both contribute in their own unique way to understanding and alleviating human suffering.

Analysing the individual stories of patients could never identify the cause of 'Pendred's syndrome' (a rare inherited disease that causes an enlarged thyroid gland and hearing loss). Making a decision between a 'thyroidectomy' (removal of the thyroid gland by surgery) and radioactive iodine (used to treat some forms of thyroid overactivity) is helped by knowledge of the effectiveness and safety of each of the two options. But that alone is not enough for making the right decision for an individual patient. Here is where the unique living experience of that person and of others that have undergone these treatments complements scientific knowledge.

Both Aristotle and Plato were in search of truth and both deserve respect. In this book, the focus is on the Aristotelian method of pursuing scientific knowledge and truth through facts and critical thinking.

Getting close to the truth through scientific knowledge requires accessing information. If you search 'thyroid' on Google, half a billion items pop up. 'Thyroid treatment' yields around 200 million hits. Advice is plentiful and comes from various sources. Some originate from medical institutions and organisations, individual healthcare professionals and patients who want to share their experience and do something good for others. Others are from hard selling profit seekers who mercilessly flog their products: books, diagnostic tests, supplements, vitamins, minerals, herbs, dubious 'online services', 'treatment plans' and 'protocols'.

This information overload is usually not a good start for someone who has been wondering about having thyroid disease, who has been diagnosed with one or for anyone who has an interest in thyroid diseases. Even when confining the search to the medical literature, the evidence can appear to be contradictory and confusing.

At the end of my last working day as a doctor, I placed my personal belongings in a cardboard box, locked the office, removed the sign with my name on the door and headed towards the lift. As I passed the window that faces the car park, the remains of the Old Infirmary that housed wards 10 and 12 caught my eye. It was where I spent many days and nights as a houseman 37 years earlier. Now its ghost was standing silent, lifeless and bare waiting for the demolition workers to put it to rest (Fig. 2). It did not feel sad. It had fulfilled its purpose and it had come to its natural finishing line, like retirement I thought.

Before the lift doors shut, two ladies in light brown 'domestics' uniforms entered. Their faces were familiar and we exchanged a cursory 'hello'. They looked at me up and down and peered into the box with my odd bits and pieces (photos of my family, some books, a small wooden carved elephant gifted by a patient from Mumbai, an old CD player and my favourite classic guitar CDs). 'My last day at work' I said. They wished me happy retirement and one asked 'What kind of doctor are you...eh...were you?' I reckoned 'endocrinologist' might complicate things, so I replied, 'I dealt with thyroid problems...' and prepared to give a short explanation. 'I know what that is!' said the other woman. 'That's when you get fat and you feel tired all the time'. I smiled as I was reminded of what I call the thyroid equation:

Getting fat + Feeling tired all the time = Thyroid trouble

The main fault of the thyroid equation is that most of the time it is wrong. For example, one study showed that hypothyroidism is present only in 4% of obese people [4], and another showed that fatigue was as common in hypothyroidism as for the rest of the population [5].

The lift had reached ground level and I walked on towards my car. Isn't it funny? I thought. Of all the possible causes of gaining weight and feeling tired, the probability of thyroid disease being the culprit is certainly not on the top of the list, yet this sample of public opinion rated it so.

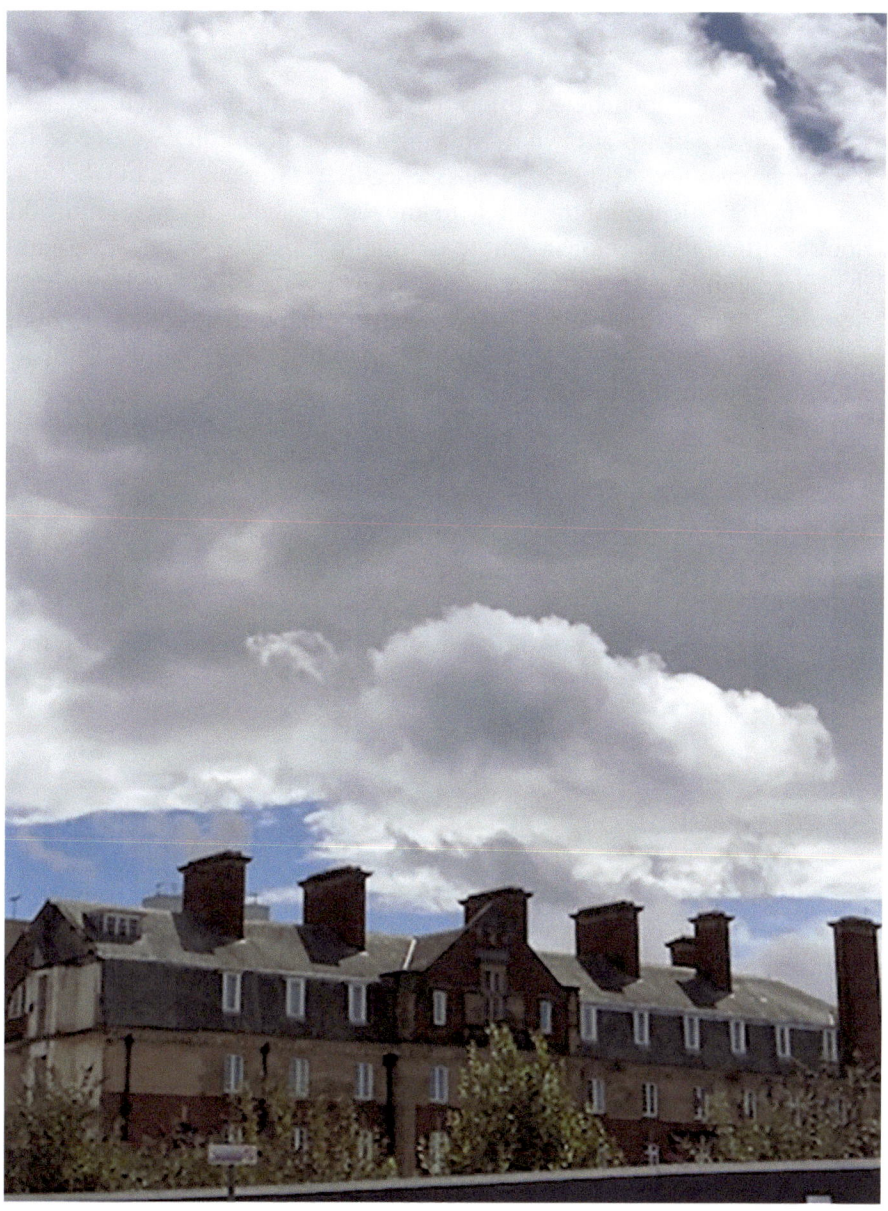

Fig. 2 The remains of the Old Victoria Wing, Royal Victoria Infirmary in Newcastle Upon Tyne (2023)

The Thyroid Equation

People are now much better informed about health than when my career started. My experience, drawn from being a junior doctor in wards 10 and 12 to exiting my office for the last time as a healthcare worker, told me that there is a desire by patients and the public to know more about the thyroid. In addition, healthcare professionals whose training has focused on practical rather than academic aspects of patient care are increasingly involved in treating thyroid patients, and they too have a need to expand their knowledge about the thyroid. Many books about the thyroid have been written aimed at patients. They tend to focus on how the thyroid gland works, how to diagnose and how to treat thyroid diseases. Some are authoritative and informative, others are instruments of misinformation. What they all have in common is that significant parts of their content become rapidly outdated as scientific evidence is evolving at an ever increasing pace.

Having listened to many thyroid patients, their carers, medical students, trainee doctors, colleagues and friends, it became apparent to me that there is a thirst for good quality, up-to-date information on the thyroid, which more often than not, fails to reach those that seek it. This was the principal reason for writing this book.

'Give a Man a Fish, You Feed Him for a Day…'

My education was what I would call 'traditional'. It consisted of learning facts, memorising dates and formulas under the austere supervision of unforgiving teachers and being able to regurgitate them under examination conditions. As I progressed in seniority through the medical ranks, the demands to teach medical students and trainees increased. When I became a father, recourse to all teaching resources became a parenting emergency.

My aversion to traditional teaching methods such as those I endured in my early life, and my experiences as a teacher of medical students, medical trainees and my own children led to one firm conclusion encapsulated by the proverb 'Give a man a fish, you feed him for a day. Teach a man to fish, you feed him for a lifetime' (Fig. 3).

If I was to write a book on the thyroid, rather than offer my interpretation of the scientific knowledge that is available, is it not better to equip people with the skills that will allow them to judge for themselves? Grasping the nuances of medical research is not an easy task, and it takes a large amount of

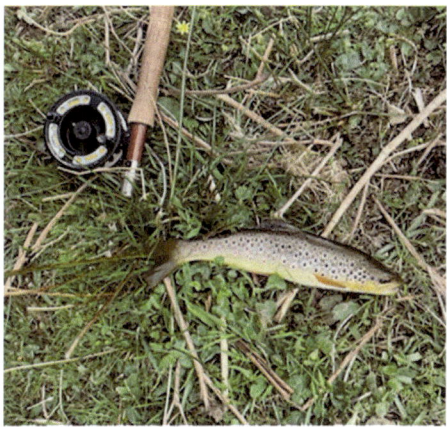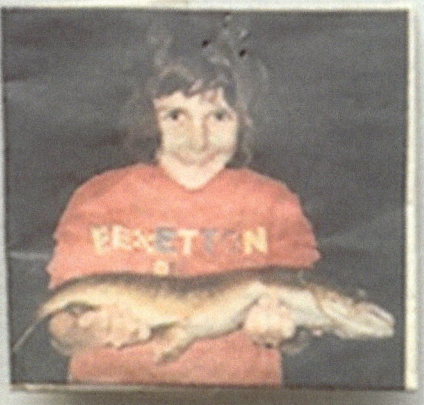

Fig. 3 'Give a man a fish, and you feed him for a day. Teach a man (or a little girl) to fish and you feed him for a lifetime'. Chinese proverb

background knowledge and experience to master it. But I have come to the conclusion that those who argue against empowering people without a PhD in health sciences, underestimate their ability. They may never acquire the same acumen as professional academics, but they can improve. And that is what this book is about, improving one's ability to get to the important sources and making better sense of it. Perhaps some guidance and sharing of useful tips can serve as catalyst to transforming superficial, hasty searches to meaningful and insightful openings that lead closer to the truth.

Aim

The aim of this book is to provide the tools that can be used to get close to the latest evidence, so that the reader (be it a patient, or anyone interested in the thyroid) has a chance to find, digest, appraise and then either embrace or reject it. No prior technical or scientific knowledge is presumed.

Layout

I have kept the book relatively short and included many pictures because I think they make reading easier. Besides, my brother Giorgos created many of the drawings with thyroid themes especially for this book, and I like them very much. I included personal anecdotes because… well, they just popped up in my head as I was writing and I hope they add some context to what is being discussed.

The book consists of three parts. 'Part I: The Basics' contains three chapters. *Chapter 1* ('Obstacles to seeking the truth') discusses the common hurdles that can come between us and the knowledge we seek, some of which are deeply embedded within our own psyche.

Chapter 2 ('Thyroid basics') is an overview of the structure and function of the thyroid gland and the common diseases that affect it, narrated through the convoluted history of discoveries relating to the thyroid. These basic facts are essential background knowledge that will help with subsequent chapters. Much of it will probably be known to many readers, but some probably not, and I hope it will be an interesting read.

Chapter 3 ('What is the evidence') discusses evidence-based medicine, how different medical publications are classified, the processes involved in publishing medical 'papers' (a 'paper' is a scientific publication, or article in a journal) and how they are structured. This is relevant and important in understanding the selection process in play that a piece of academic work is subjected to before it reaches its readers, how it varies and how it may correlate with the quality of the end product.

'Part II: The Manual' consists of *Chaps. 4–6*. Two of these (*Chaps. 5 and 6*) contain checklists and the reader can come back to these chapters when faced with a particular question or paper and look up the steps that can lead to the answers.

Chapter 4 ('Mining the truth') is about conducting searches. It identifies appropriate search engines and gives tips on how to stay on course. A key message to patients is don't do this entirely by yourself.

Chapter 5 ('Appraising the evidence') outlines how to judge the quality of published papers based on checklists.

Chapter 6 ('Interpreting the evidence') will help extract the meaning of a piece of research. This was the hardest part to write because of the complexity of this process. The ability to judge evidence evolves with experience and practice, so it takes effort and time. *Chapter 6* provides some of the basic rules that can be used to develop and build upon this skill.

'Part III: An Opinion' is an example of a common question asked by patients with hypothyroidism (the commonest thyroid condition). It will reveal a truth that should be making headlines and attracting the attention of patient advocates, thyroid specialists, their professional organisations and the public at large. Yet all relevant parties seem to choose to ignore it and channel their energies in other directions. It is an example of good science yielding valuable knowledge, which is undermined and made worthless by poor implementation. Herein lies the most important message of this book: seeking truth and getting close to it is not enough, how it is used to change the lives of patients is what really matters.

I have included a lexicon for the technical terms encountered and relevant bibliography at the end of each chapter to indicate the sources in case the reader wishes to access them.

References

1. Smith SM, Zwart SR, McMonigal KA, Huntoon CL. Thyroid status of space shuttle crewmembers: effects of iodine removal. Aviat Space Environ Med. 2011;82(1):49–51. https://doi.org/10.3357/asem.2926.2011.
2. Innocenti C, Fioravanti G, Spiti R, Faravelli C. [The Stendhal syndrome between psychoanalysis and neuroscience]. Riv Psichiatr. 2014;49(2):61–6. La sindrome di Stendhal fra psicoanalisi e neuroscienze. https://doi.org/10.1708/1461.16139.
3. School of Athens. https://en.wikipedia.org/wiki/File:%22The_School_of_Athens%22_by_Raffaello_Sanzio_da_Urbino.jpg.
4. Mahdavi M, Amouzegar A, Mehran L, Madreseh E, Tohidi M, Azizi F. Investigating the prevalence of primary thyroid dysfunction in obese and overweight individuals: Tehran thyroid study. BMC Endocr Disord. 2021;21(1):89. https://doi.org/10.1186/s12902-021-00743-4.
5. van de Ven AC, Netea-Maier RT, de Vegt F, et al. Is there a relationship between fatigue perception and the serum levels of thyrotropin and free thyroxine in euthyroid subjects? Thyroid. 2012;22(12):1236–43. https://doi.org/10.1089/thy.2011.0200.

Contents

Part III   An Opinion

Author and Illustrator

About the Author

Petros Perros studied Physiology and Biochemistry before becoming a doctor. He specialised in endocrinology and practised as thyroid specialist for 27 years in Newcastle upon Tyne, UK. He was a founding member, secretary and president of the European Group on Graves' Orbitopathy. He is patron of the British Thyroid Foundation and has served as medical advisor for several other thyroid patient organisations. He published more than 200 peer-reviewed academic papers and 21 book chapters, mostly on thyroid topics. He lectured as invited speaker in many national and international academic meetings. He is currently Visiting Senior Lecturer at Newcastle University having retired from clinical practice in 2021.

About the Illustrator

Giorgos Perros is a mathematician and an artist. He studied mathematics and mathematical logic in Newcastle upon Tyne and London. He taught mathematics for 35 years at Anatolia College, Thessaloniki, Greece.

Part I

The Basics

1

Obstacles to Seeking Truth

'Trust and admiration for a person are no guarantee that their views are true'

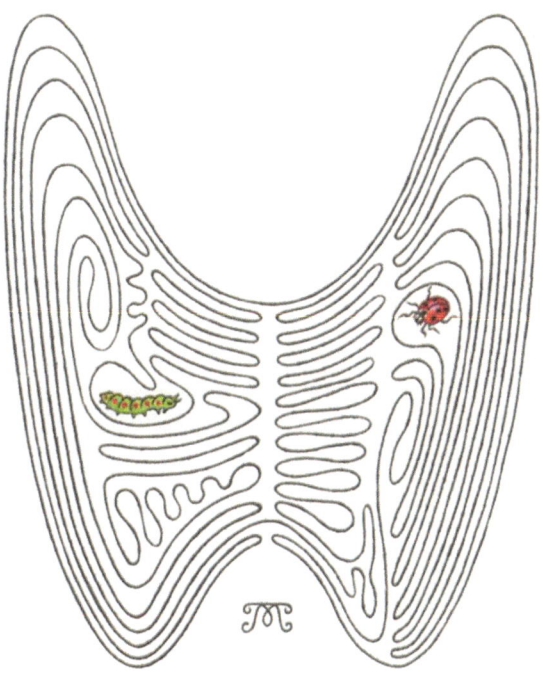

Some truths about the thyroid are simple, like its shape which looks like a butterfly. Others require you to go hunting in a maze full of dead ends and diversions. But the rewards for finding truth are as great as those of a hungry ladybird's feast on a caterpillar

Brace Yourself

Before you start your search for the truth about the thyroid, you need to be prepared to face reality. For every bit of treasure, there will be heaps of irrelevant and distracting trash. Get ready to defend yourself by recognising some of the common traps. I learned my first lesson about truth many years ago, and I have Uncle Alekos to thank for it.

The Truth According to Uncle Alekos

I grew up in a small town in northern Greece surrounded by dozens of uncles, aunts and cousins. Many of my relatives dropped in unannounced for a 'kouvenda' (a chat and catching up, always spiced with some gossip). For me, one of the most welcome visitors was Uncle Alekos. This chain-smoking, willowy, Humphrey Bogart look-alike was no ordinary man (Fig. 1.1). During the German occupation of World War II, he joined the partisans in the mountains. In the turmoil that followed the German retreat, civil war broke out in 1946. Uncle Alekos sided with the Stalin-inspired communists. His older

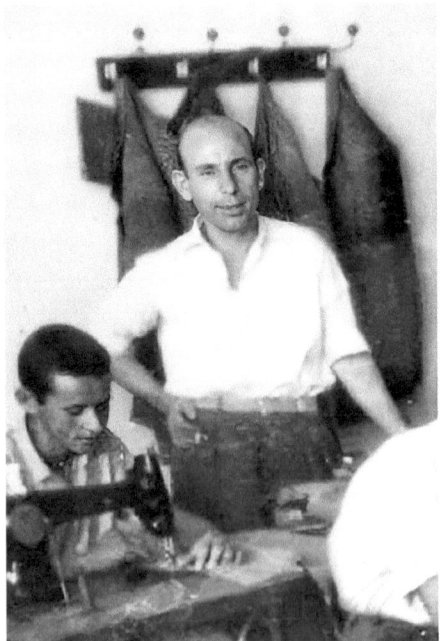

Fig. 1.1 Uncle Alekos in his workshop

brother Takis, a law student, was a leading Trotskyist. Uncle Alekos was present at a communist committee meeting when a decision was made that several men and women from our town were 'enemies of the people', among them his brother. He warned Takis and urged him to hide. Takis ignored his brother's advice, disappeared soon after and was never seen again. Alekos's uncle, an eminent doctor in the area with liberal political inclinations, had a similar fate.

Uncle Alekos was not educated other than in the 'University of Life' as he called it. He endured poverty and discrimination because of his political past. Eventually, he settled down, became a tailor and raised a family.

His visits to our home were eagerly welcomed by the matriarch in our family, my grandmother and aunt of Alekos. Her curriculum vitae included losing her husband and her 19-year-old daughter within a year of each other when she was barely 40 years old. Somehow she survived the misery of bereavement, destitution and the burden of bringing up two younger children, among them my mother.

Despite the hardships that life had handed out to Uncle Alekos and my grandmother, these were two people with the most admirable optimism that I have ever known. Uncle Alekos's visits were always welcome. He would sit cross-legged and slowly light an unfiltered cigarette. A small cup of steaming sweet coffee with a creamy head and muddy sediment would be served accompanied by an ice-cold glass of water and a spoonful of home-made glazed bergamot delicately placed on a small crystal plate with a tiny spoon before the 'kouvenda' got going.

The conversation would meander around the past, the present and the future with no discernible pattern involving people, events local and international, stories and anecdotes, hearsay and, of course, some gossip (neither clergy nor relatives and friends were spared).

Invariably Uncle Alekos would express one or more of his strong opinions on some important matter. Be it the upcoming mayoral elections, the Cold War or the landing on the moon, Uncle Alekos would state his conclusions, which ranged from interesting to preposterous. And he had the most powerful argument to support his views. His voice would drop a semitone and his rhythm would slow by a fraction, he would lean slightly forward and look you straight in the eye: 'listen to what Alekos is telling you', and he would utter his views with supreme conviction, implying that he had exclusive access to absolute truths.

I am reminded of Uncle Alekos every time I am tempted to believe something because a person or a source I respect says so. Uncle Alekos' views, though entertaining, colourful, mostly harmless and seemingly credible, were just opinions and were rather short on truth. I owe it to Uncle Alekos for learning that the source of information (though important) is not sufficient in the quest for truth.

Bias, the Ubiquitous Enemy

In medical research, typically a treatment or drug is tested on a population of patients, and the results are collected and then analysed. The conclusion may be that a treatment is beneficial. Then an assumption is made that because the treatment worked in the sample of patients tested, it must also work in all patients with the same condition. When the doctor prescribes that treatment to a patient, a further assumption is made, that the particular patient will respond in the same way as the majority. Key to this is whether the original population of patients tested was truly representative of the whole and whether the individual patient to be treated is sufficiently similar to the majority. Given how we differ from each other in age, sex, genetic makeup, lifestyle and numerous other characteristics, the scope for the transition from experimental evidence to treating a patient in real life being derailed is significant.

After seat belts were introduced in cars in the 1960s, it became evident that women suffered disproportionate injuries and deaths from car accidents compared to men, despite wearing seat belts. It turned out that early seat belt designs were based on the size of an average man [1]. The underlying assumption was that all drivers were men and that, if you are a driver, the particular seat belt design (based on the build of an average man) is right for you.

Bias is everywhere and often catches us unaware. Scientists need to be constantly mindful of bias when conducting their research. If one is to appraise the evidence fairly, then there is a need to be aware of and look out for bias.

Cromwell's Rule and Popper's Swans

In 1650 [2], Oliver Cromwell addressed the General Assembly of the Church of Scotland and asked them to reconsider their theological position. He included the phrase '*I beseech you, in the bowels of Christ, think it possible that you may be mistaken*'. It has become known as 'Cromwell's rule' in statistics and highlights that however small a probability may be, it should not be completely ignored. Cromwell's rule is a reminder that our preconceived ideas and beliefs must not be unshakeable. If convincing evidence arrives that is contrary to our beliefs, we must be prepared to accept it.

Sir Karl Popper dedicated a large part of his life to studying the methods that scientists use. He challenged conventional thinking by proposing that rather than trying to prove a theory right, scientists should try to prove it wrong [3]. Popper's famous swan argument states that if we believe that all swans are white, then the only way of verifying it is to observe all the swans on earth, an almost impossible task. On the other hand, if one single black swan is observed, our theory is overturned.

Being deeply entrenched in our own unshaken beliefs, unable and unwilling to even entertain the possibility that we may be wrong and striving to prove right the answer we want are common obstacles to finding truth.

Rooster Syndrome and Kahneman's Systems One and Two

Imagine that you were born and raised on a farm and grew up without any contact with the outside world. Every morning the cockerel crowed before the sun rose. Having observed this sequence thousands of times, would it not be tempting to assume that it is the cockerel's crow that makes the sun rise? This tendency to assume causation when one event is linked with another is an error that we all make.

Daniel Kahneman (who started as a psychologist and ended up winning the Nobel prize in economics) refers to two kinds of thinking that go on in the human brain. 'System One' is a fast-reacting process that depends on past experiences and emotions [4]. 'System Two' is the deeper thinker within us, slower and analytical. System One tends to regard associations as being causally related. We can thank System One for the survival of our primitive ancestors, who reacted instinctively to the faintest of sounds of an approaching predator, for such a warning system has to be sensitive and inevitably results in false alarms. In today's world, most of the challenges and choices we make need a System Two approach, but we are still often ruled by the rooster syndrome and System One [5].

Illusory Truth Effect

'*Repeat a lie often enough and it becomes the truth*' is a phrase attributed to Joseph Goebbels. Lies about Jewish people convinced an entire nation. Experimental evidence shows that simply reading or listening to a statement like '*an elephant weighs less than an ant*' makes us more likely to believe it [6].

This is the 'illusory truth effect', well described in psychology [7] and taken advantage of by advertisers, politicians and those that like to spread misinformation. Of course, it does not necessarily follow that every bit of repeated information is false but the fact that a view is popular does not necessarily make it credible.

Quality Not Quantity

Back in 2014, I received an email from a sender that I did not recognise with the message: '*Someone recently sent me a link to your article (….) and I thought you might be interested in my research. I've done an exhaustive study of thyroid physiology, and I think you might find some of the concepts presented in my book intriguing*'. She went on '*My book has over 900 references and I know you will enjoy it if you're truly interested in thyroid physiology*'.

Being somewhat of a sceptic, I surmised that this author (probably urged by her publisher) sent this same email to lots of other random people as part of her promotional campaign. I replied that I did not feel I was in need of this book and that I normally relied on reading the 'peer-reviewed' medical literature ('peer review' is a process whereby independent experts in the field scrutinise and approve scientific writings before they are published). It was the beginning of several email exchanges during the course of which she tried to persuade me to order a copy of her book and repeated at every opportunity her mantra that her book contained 900 references.

I have resisted reading her book to this day because judging from some of the claims made in her emails and some extracts that I have seen, I was uninspired. My own biases admittedly may have also prevailed. The 900 references were supposed to impress and lend credence to her opinions.

Like many other commodities, quality rather than quantity trips this type of argument. Simply the number of references or words or pictures in a book or article by itself can be an unreliable metric. Watson and Crick's publication on the structure of DNA in 1953 was to propel biology and medicine into the most amazing discoveries of the twentieth and twenty-first centuries. It contained only six references.8

The Devil Is in the Detail

A few years ago, I led a seminar for trainees in *Endocrinology* during which appraisal of the medical literature was discussed. I projected on the screen the title of a paper that has been cited hundreds of times since its publication, as evidence that patients with 'hypothyroidism' who are treated with levothyroxine (a medicine that is identical to the missing hormone in hypothyroid patients) are more prone to experiencing persistent symptoms compared to the background population, even when their thyroid blood tests are normal [9].

My question to the trainees was which section of the paper was most important. The options were abstract (summary), introduction, methods, results, discussion and conclusions. The least popular choice was the methods. This is not surprising as the methods section is the most boring part of any paper and medical papers are generally pretty dull. However, if one wishes to judge the quality of a paper, the methods section is vital.

One critical piece of information in the methods of this particular paper was how participants were chosen. It turns out that they were picked for being prescribed levothyroxine by their family doctor, which (the devil is in the detail) may not necessarily be the same as having been diagnosed with hypothyroidism. More of this later.

Ready to Go

So, beware of opinions that are based on opinions, people who are never wrong, mind illusory ants and elephants, think of quality, not quantity, look out for the devil in the detail, use your System Two, and you will be fine.

References

1. Criado-Perez C. Invisible women. Penguin; 2019.
2. Cromwell O. To the general assembly of the Kirk of Scotland. https://www.oliver-cromwell.org/Letters_and_speeches/letters/Letter_129.pdf.
3. Popper K. The logic of scientific discovery. Routledge; 2002.
4. Kahneman D. Thinking, fast and slow. Farrar, Straus and Giroux; 2011.
5. Gould SJ. The mismeasure of man. WW Norton & Co; 1996.
6. Fazio LK, Rand DG, Pennycook G. Repetition increases perceived truth equally for plausible and implausible statements. Psychon Bull Rev. 2019;26(5):1705–10. https://doi.org/10.3758/s13423-019-01651-4.
7. Hassan A, Barber SJ. The effects of repetition frequency on the illusory truth effect. Cogn Res Princ Implic. 2021;6(1):38. https://doi.org/10.1186/s41235-021-00301-5.
8. Watson JD, Crick FH. Molecular structure of nucleic acids; a structure for deoxyribose nucleic acid. Nature. 1953;171(4356):737–8. https://doi.org/10.1038/171737a0.
9. Saravanan P, Chau WF, Roberts N, Vedhara K, Greenwood R, Dayan CM. Psychological well-being in patients on 'adequate' doses of l-thyroxine: results of a large, controlled community-based questionnaire study. Clin Endocrinol (Oxf). 2002;57(5):577–85. https://doi.org/10.1046/j.1365-2265.2002.01654.x.

2

Thyroid Basics

‘Everything about the thyroid gland is delicate, complicated, synchronised and in perfect harmony…’

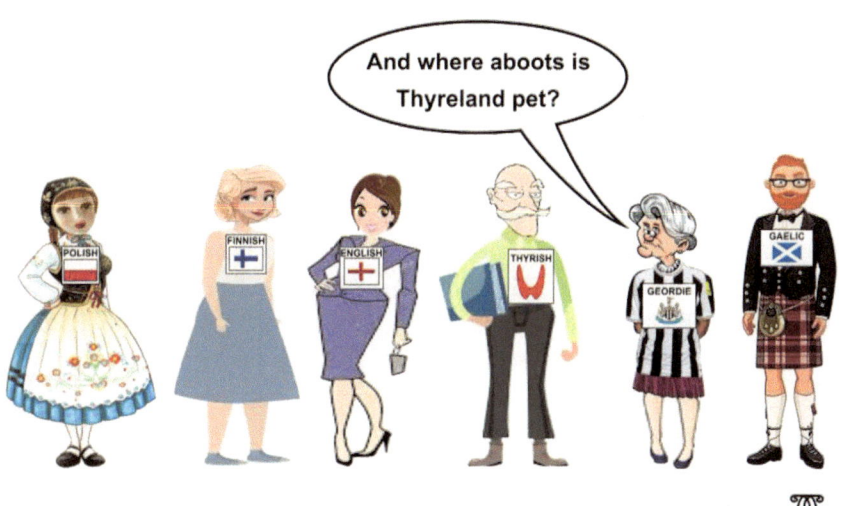

P. Perros, *Seeking Thyroid Truths*, Copernicus Books,
https://doi.org/10.1007/978-3-031-58287-5_2

A Historical Perspective

Our knowledge of the thyroid has a long history full of blind alleys, cul-de-sacs, prejudices, failures and occasional triumphs. Today, we are in a position to replace and manipulate the function of the thyroid gland in numerous ways. We can also wipe it out with drugs, surgery, laser, heat, radiation and even alcohol injections. This has been possible because of the knowledge that accumulated over thousands of years through observations, study and experimentation. Understanding where we have got to requires some familiarity with the structure and function of the thyroid gland. Approaching thyroid basics through history illustrates how elusive truth can be, how hard it is to gain knowledge and how easily we can be misled. It is also a way of understanding where many terms and names relating to the thyroid came from.

The story of the thyroid has its origins in the formation of the oceans four billion years ago. Iodine (one of the basic elements of the material world) washed out of the mountains and plains into the seas, where life began. But before delving into all that, let me introduce you to 'Thyrish'.

Do You Speak 'Thyrish'?

A few years into my consultant post, I met Mrs. S who came to my clinic accompanied by her husband. The pair of them were highly anxious and as soon as Mrs. S sat down, she handed me a letter and said: '*I have read everything that's in there doctor, but I cannot understand a word. It must be very serious*'. They had been on holiday in Florida, where she became ill and ended up in hospital. This resulted in many tests, no treatment and a four-figure bill. She was advised that she was safe to travel home and that she must see an endocrinologist as soon as possible.

The letter was written and signed by a US board-certified endocrinologist. It read: *Mrs. S presented to the ER with anterior cervical pain and sinus tachycardia. She gave a past history of post-partum thyroiditis. Investigations showed a suppressed thyroid-stimulating hormone (TSH), high normal total T4 and normal T3, TPO antibodies were elevated, TRAb marginally above range, thyroid uptake scintigram low-normal uptake, CRP and ESR minimally elevated. Diagnosis: subclinical hyperthyroidism due to Graves' disease/Hashitoxicosis/De Quervain thyroiditis. Suggest repeat TFTs and inflammatory markers, consider adding TSI*.

'Thyrish' is a language that has evolved over many years. It is spoken fluently only by trained endocrinologists, who are required to attain a Certificate of Advanced Thyrish issued after competency is reached, by passing an exam set by their professional body. It consists of abbreviations, eponyms, acronyms, and words derived from ancient Greek, Latin and a combination of the two.

The intention is to enable endocrinologists to communicate with each other in code and to instil an aura of mystical supremacy over non-Thyrish speakers. Thyrish was designed to be incomprehensible by the lay public and even other medical specialists who tend to be perplexed and irritated by it. One alleged reason why Thyrish is still popular among endocrinologists is the joy that it brings upon them when observing the bemusement of colleagues in other specialties (especially surgeons) when Thyrish is spoken.

I will strive to translate Thyrish words immediately as they are encountered in this book. In addition, you will find a Thyrish-English Lexicon at the very end of the book.

The text in the letter that Mrs. S brought to my clinic will not be translated in order to create a sense of suspense; however, the answers can be found in the Thyrish-English Lexicon should the curiosity of impatient readers prevail.

What Is the Thyroid?

The thyroid is an 'endocrine gland' located in the neck. A 'gland' is an organ that produces secretions. The salivary glands produce saliva, the lacrimal glands tears, the pancreas digestive juices as well as several hormones, with insulin being the most important. 'Endocrine' means that the products of a gland are released into the bloodstream rather than to a particular part of the body outside the circulation (called 'exocrine'). The salivary glands are exocrine because they release saliva into the mouth, and the thyroid gland is endocrine because it releases its products into the bloodstream.

The products of endocrine glands are 'hormones' or chemical messages that use the circulation as a highway to reach other parts of the body and deliver instructions. Lymph nodes are also sometimes referred to as 'glands', although they serve different functions related to the immune system rather than making hormones. This sometimes causes confusion because we happen to have lots of lymph nodes around the thyroid gland, and lymph nodes in the neck often become enlarged and sometimes painful due to infections.

Celeb Neck

On a thyroid patient website, a picture of a celebrity (who has sadly since passed away) was posted (Fig. 2.1), drawing attention to a 'lump' in the celeb's neck. Fellow bloggers were quick to respond and agreed that she was in great need of thyroid help.

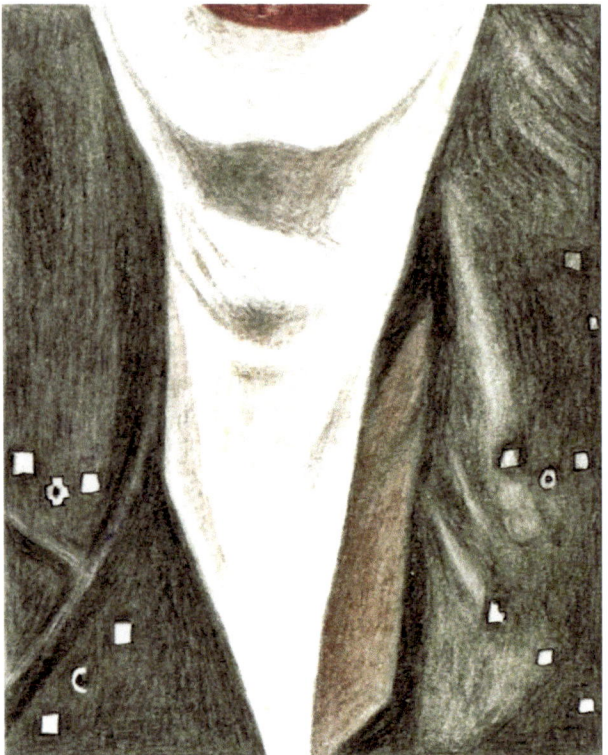

Fig. 2.1 Celeb neck

One who could not spot the problem was duly guided to the abnormality in the neck and replied that she could now see the obvious lump, how could she have missed it before?

Among the 26 exchanges, there was one sceptic who thought that the lump in the neck was Adam's apple but was quickly silenced by the majority. Most agreed that the breast cancer, which the unfortunate celeb was known to suffer from, had spread to her thyroid. The question that arose next among discussants was whether someone should tell her, maybe through Twitter. Eventually the consensus that prevailed was that she had enough on her plate with her stage 4 breast cancer and she probably would have been checked for thyroid anyway; therefore, it is best to let it rest.

It is astonishing how poorly the anatomy of the neck is understood by doctors, never mind lay people, and how bad doctors can be at examining the neck. During my working life as an endocrinologist, I regularly received referrals about patients with 'lumps in the thyroid'. In roughly 50% of the cases when the patient was asked to indicate where the lump was, they pointed to areas in the neck that were not the thyroid (usually the Adam's apple).

Sometimes when doctors are uncertain of what they are feeling in the neck, rather than brush up on their examination skills, they send patients for an ultrasound examination. From then onwards, it is downhill all the way because about 50% of middle-aged or older people have at least one small thyroid lump if examined with an ultrasound scan.

If one starts to investigate people's thyroid glands who have no symptoms arising from their thyroid (like the celeb), we can end up performing invasive tests like biopsies (taking a sample of tissue for examination). In a significant proportion of cases, this escalates to a thyroid operation (because the biopsy in about a quarter of the cases does not provide a clear answer), just in case there is an underlying cancer. This trend, unfortunately, has spread like wildfire in several countries, mainly rich ones [1]. Having lived through this epidemic over the past 20 years, the lesson learned is that in most cases, it is more harmful to investigate people who have no symptoms for possible thyroid lumps than not [2].

The Anatomy of the Thyroid Gland

If you run a finger perpendicularly downwards starting from the midline from under the chin (Fig. 2.2), about a third of the way down the neck you will feel something hard. This is the top of the 'thyroid cartilage'. If you feel up and down and sideways at this point, you will notice a notch, which confirms that you are at the upper border of the thyroid cartilage. The thyroid cartilage is

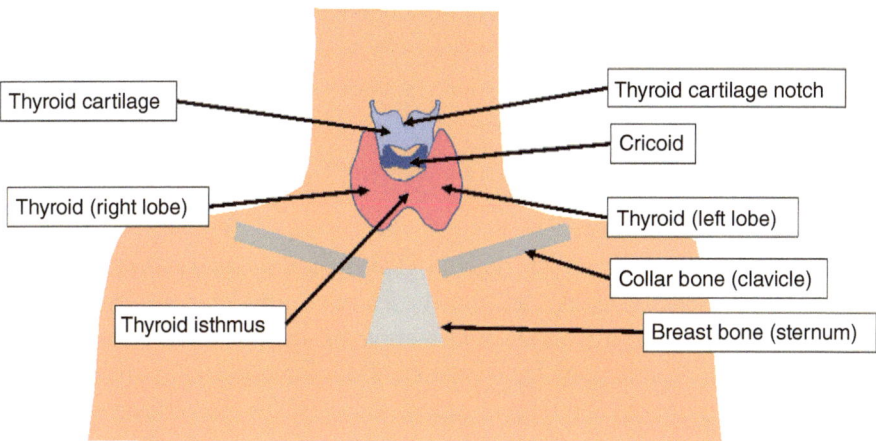

Fig. 2.2 Position of the thyroid gland in the neck and surrounding landmarks

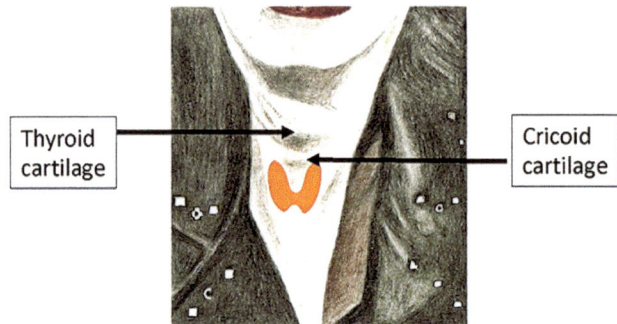

Fig. 2.3 Position of the thyroid and cricoid cartilages. The thyroid gland (shown in orange) lies below the cricoid cartilage and is not visible

not part of the thyroid (it is called so because it is near the thyroid). Then continue to run your finger down (Fig. 2.2) and you will immediately feel a thin, horizontal, hard bump. This is the 'cricoid cartilage'. This too is not part of the thyroid gland. If you then feel a little further down, the tissues are soft (Fig. 2.2), and you are now at the central part of the thyroid gland (called the 'isthmus') that joins the right with the left sides of the thyroid.

Immediately below the isthmus is where the collar bones meet the breastbone. The two main parts of the thyroid gland (the right and left 'lobes') are connected to the isthmus and normally cannot be seen or felt unless they are enlarged.

Take another look at the celeb's picture (Fig. 2.3), and you will appreciate that what drew the attention of bloggers was her prominent Adam's apple (thyroid and cricoid cartilage), a normal feature especially in people with thin necks. Her thyroid gland was sitting below the cricoid cartilage (shown in orange in Fig. 2.3) and that part of her neck is completely flat.

What Does the Thyroid Do?

Historical Clues

The earliest description of the thyroid gland (though it was not called so for another 100 years) was in 1543 by the Flemish physician Andeas Vesalius, who was particularly interested in human anatomy, but what the thyroid did would not become known for centuries. This did not prevent plentiful and colourful opinions [3]. In the seventeenth century Thomas Wharton, an anatomist who coined the term 'thyroid' (meaning shield in ancient Greek), wrote a book on glands entitled *'Adenographia: sive glandularum totius corporis descriptio'* (Adenographia: or the description of the glands of the entire body)

[4]. On page 111 he wrote, '*The thyroid contributes much to round and beautify the neck, fills the empty spaces around the larynx, and smooths and flattens parts of its protuberances, particularly in women where it is larger for this very reason and adds uniformity and charm to their necks*'.

In the seventeenth century, medicine as a healing profession was still in its infancy. Physicians were obsessed with studying the structure of the human body, and they were meticulously observant. But attempts to guess the function of the different parts were most often highly inaccurate and heavily influenced by the belief that the Almighty had built humans with a purpose. So, the function had to be understood in the context of divinity. And here came all kinds of biases, including the outrageous idea that the purpose of the thyroid was to beautify the neck, 'particularly in women' [4, 5]. Wharton's contribution was limited to inventing the term 'thyroid'. His ideas about the function of the thyroid did not make contribute to his fame.

In 1806, Rush (an eminent American physician, politician, co-signatory of the Declaration of Independence and founder of American Psychiatry) wrote that the function of the thyroid gland is to '*defend the brain from the morbid effects of all the causes which determine the blood into it, with unusual force*' [6]. He went on to explain that the larger thyroid gland in women as being '*necessary to guard the female system from the influence of the more numerous causes of irritation and vexation of mind to which they are exposed than the male sex*'. These distractions were not only deeply misogynistic and unhelpful but also misleading and did anything but advance knowledge. Recent studies on the size of the thyroid glands of normal men and women, using ultrasound, show the opposite. Men have a slightly larger thyroid gland than women [7]. The seventeenth-to-nineteenth-century belief that women had larger thyroid glands than men was probably due to errors in measurements, lack of understanding the precise anatomy of the thyroid gland or too few individuals being studied.

The understanding of the function of the thyroid came from four main sources:

- Observations relating to conditions that occurred naturally, especially 'goitre' (enlargement of the thyroid gland), 'cretinism' (a devastating condition affecting infants that lead to mental and growth retardation) and 'myxoedema' (severe underactivity of the thyroid)
- Advances in surgery for safe removal of goitres and the observation that removal of the thyroid frequently led to these patients developing myxoedema
- Discovery of iodine
- A peculiar vogue developed in the nineteenth century for 'organotherapy', that is, injection of mushed up organs into patients as treatments for a variety of diseases

Goitre was recognised more than 2000 years ago and was treated with seaweed in China [8]. This was the first clue that one cause of goitre ('endemic' goitre) is the lack of a substance contained in seaweed, now known to be iodine. This knowledge probably did not influence progress in Western Medicine in relation to the function of the thyroid. However, endemic goitre was common in Europe and in most parts of the world. So, doctors were familiar with it for many centuries before the function of the thyroid was known.

'Endemic' means that a disease is confined to certain geographical areas, in contrast to a 'pandemic' that we are all familiar with implying that a disease is widespread. It was also known that endemic goitre was common in mountainous areas like the Alps, central Asia, central Africa and the Andes. In addition, endemic goitre was found in inland non-mountainous regions (like in Derbyshire, an area of endemic goitre in England in the past, where the term 'Derbyshire neck' was used to describe endemic goitre). Conversely, endemic goitre was rare in coastal areas. This was a clue that the place where people lived had something to do with endemic goitre and that most likely there was something in the environment that caused it.

Another important hint about the function of the thyroid gland was that cretinism was found in the same areas as endemic goitre. Indeed, children with cretinism often also had a goitre. The term 'cretin' is now used synonymously with 'stupid', 'idiot' or 'imbecile', but it comes from 'crestin', meaning Christian in an alpine dialect. It is thought that the term was used to remind people that although cretins were different and unusual, they were still human and children of Christ and deserved to be treated kindly [9]. It is odd that such a heart-warming story has been forgotten and replaced by the negative connotations that the word 'cretin' has today.

William Gull (an eminent English physician) described the features of what we now know was hypothyroidism in adults and noted some similarities with cretinism in 1874. So here was a pattern emerging that linked a collection of features (those of hypothyroidism) with a condition that affected children (cretinism) and with endemic goitre.

Four years later, William Ord (an English surgeon) published a paper describing hypothyroidism and coined the term 'myxoedema', meaning swelling due to mucus [10]. Severe, long-standing hypothyroidism makes tissues puffy due to accumulation of sticky fluid. This can be seen especially in the face, particularly around the eyes. The words 'myxoedema' and 'hypothyroidism' are sometimes used synonymously, but myxoedema usually signifies severe and long-standing, untreated hypothyroidism.

Ord described adult patients with myxoedema, who had been previously healthy without an obvious trigger. In the meantime, 700 miles away a Swiss surgeon, Emil Theodor Kocher had become famous for his good surgical results of thyroidectomies (removal of thyroid glands) of patients with endemic goitre, who were plentiful in Switzerland. But soon enough (in 1883), Kocher noticed that many of his patients developed myxoedema post-operatively. This suggested that the thyroid gland made substances whose absence caused myxoedema, a condition which happened to be identical to what Ord had described to occur spontaneously in some people.

In 1811, iodine was discovered by Bernard Courtois (Fig. 2.4). This led to its use almost indiscriminately for any disease possible including endemic goitre. Overenthusiasm led to use of massive doses of iodine, which caused serious side effects. Despite some success in treating endemic goitre, iodine treatment was discredited and abandoned [11]. Nonetheless, this detour in the quest to understand the function of the thyroid was consistent with the notion that endemic goitre was caused by iodine deficiency.

Science and medicine progress in small, tedious steps that every now and then are substituted by leaps. In 1891, George Murray, a physician who was born, educated and practiced in Newcastle upon Tyne, used an extract of sheep thyroid glands to treat a patient with myxoedema [12]. This was not exactly an inspiration that revealed itself to Murray out of thin air. 'Organotherapy' (injecting mushed up organs of animals into patients) was popular at the time, especially in continental Europe.

A year before Murray's use of thyroid extract, Charles-Edouard Brown-Séquard, a famous neurologist, claimed that injection of a fluid prepared from the testicles of animals into humans was an elixir for rejuvenation and longevity. This did not convince many of his peers in Paris and elsewhere and provoked some ridicule. Murray will have been aware of the fact that thyroidectomy was often followed by myxoedema and organotherapy, so the idea of infusing thyroid extract to patients with myxoedema was not so outlandish.

Murray's application of organotherapy to myxoedema was accompanied by evidence of symptoms and signs of myxoedema disappearing. However, he too was met by scepticism and even scorn by his fellow English physicians. The test of truth in science and medicine is reproducibility, so doubters were soon silenced by the obvious success of this new treatment. The cure for hypothyroidism had arrived, and the message spread rapidly.

By the beginning of the twentieth century, it was known that the thyroid, through substances that it released into the bloodstream, controlled body temperature and metabolism and that it affected the heart, brain, bones and in fact every organ in the body. It had also become known that the thyroid needed iodine to produce its secretions and that iodine deficiency was the cause of endemic goitre and cretinism.

We now know that the thyroid gland produces a number of hormones. The most important ones are thyroxine (also known as T4) and tri-iodothyronine

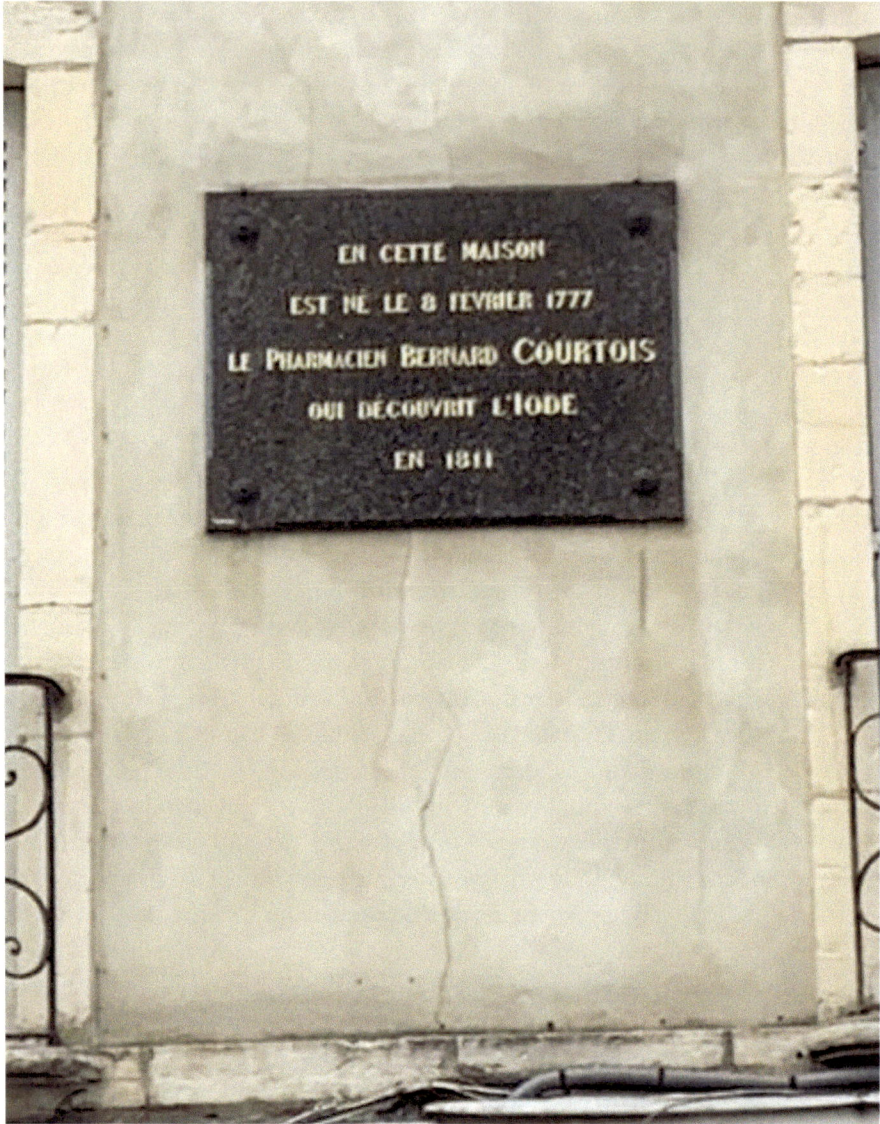

Fig. 2.4 The house of Bernard Courtois in Dijon. (Photograph courtesy of George Priestley)

(T3). Synthetically made T3, which is sometimes used for the treatment of thyroid underactivity, is referred to as liothyronine, although chemically tri-iodothyronine, liothyronine and T3 are the same. The thyroid also makes a hormone called calcitonin (involved in bone metabolism) and another compound called 3-iodothyronamine, whose role at present is unclear [13].

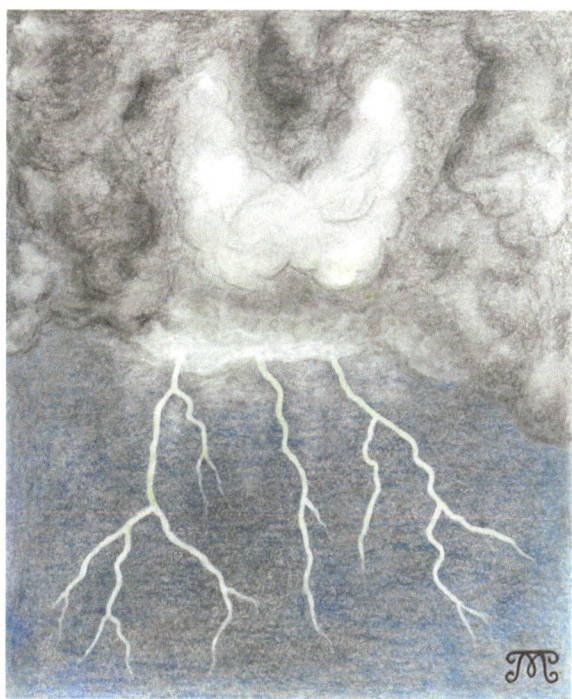

The thyroid tale has its roots in the formation of the mountains and the oceans. Storms and rainfall washed iodine into the seas, where life began. The survival of primitive organisms relied on iodine and this led to the creation of the thyroid gland

Why Iodine?

If you are designing an organ that produces hormones, why choose it to depend so heavily on a trace element like iodine and expose the organism to the risks of deficiency? It turns out that to answer this question, we need to go way back in our evolutionary history.

About three billion years ago, primitive microorganisms ('cyanobacteria') started to use 'photosynthesis' (capture the sun's energy and use it to produce and release oxygen into the atmosphere). A crucial problem that arose was the high levels of oxygen 'radicals' generated inside cells by photosynthesis. Oxygen radicals are an unstable version of oxygen that, if left unchecked, react with surrounding chemicals including DNA, lipid membranes (the outer wall of cells, as well as the lining of other important structures within cells) and other vital compounds and structures inside the cell and cause damage.

Oxygen radicals had to be neutralised by other chemicals, called 'antioxidants' [14–16]. One such antioxidant, which was plentiful within the sea environment where these creatures lived, was iodine. Over millions of years, iodine had washed out of mountains and plains into the seas, so iodine was, and still is, abundant in coastal areas; therefore, it was an obvious part of the solution (Fig. 2.5).

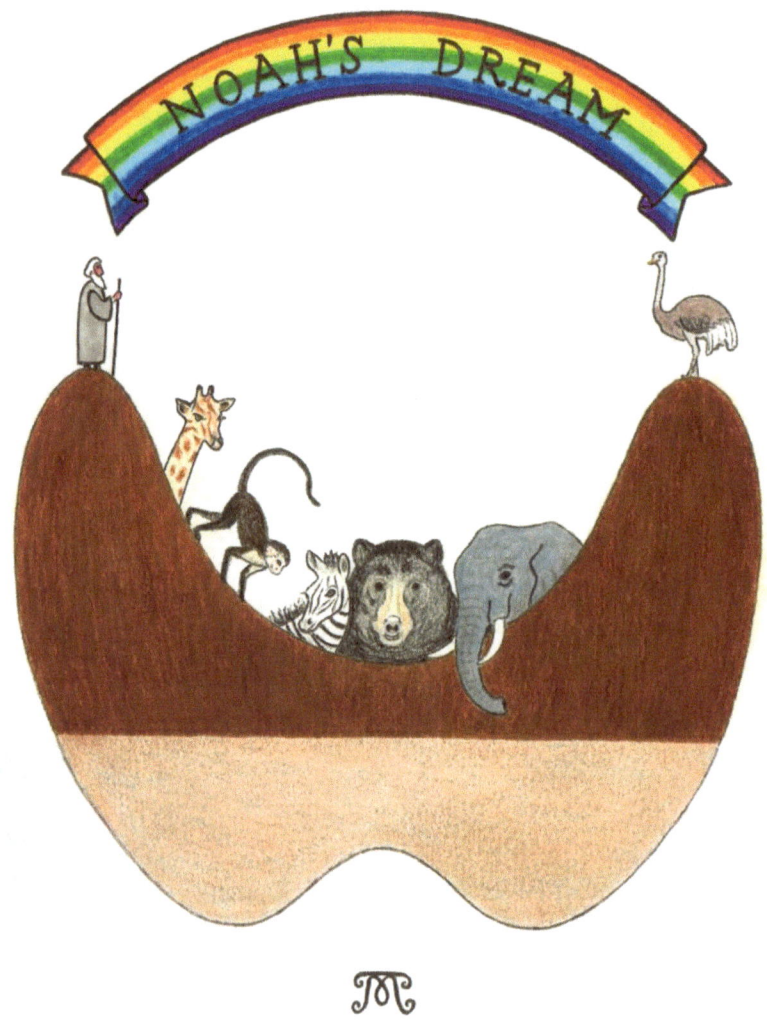

Fig. 2.5 The biblical story of the deluge is a reminder of the forces of nature that led to iodine being washed out of mountains and inland plains into coasted regions, which set the scene for the evolution of the thyroid

The chemical reactions that eliminated harmful oxygen radicals produced other iodine-rich chemical compounds that were the ancestors of thyroid hormones. Cyanobacteria were full of such iodine-containing compounds. More advanced life forms fed on cyanobacteria and grew from larvae to adult forms. For this transformation (called 'metamorphosis') to take place, enough energy stores had to be secured; otherwise, the larvae did not survive the high energy demands of metamorphosis.

The levels of iodine-rich chemicals (primitive thyroid hormones) that accumulated in the bodies of larvae mirrored how well the larvae had fed, and therefore, they served as a signal that enough energy had been stored for metamorphosis to begin. As animals evolved to more complex forms, they became capable of making thyroid hormones themselves, rather than relying on outside sources, and to use them as a way of sending signals to different tissues in the body. Besides being regulators of metabolism (Fig. 2.6), thyroid hormones have retained their ancestral role to control growth and development from juvenile to adult forms (Fig. 2.7), and cretinism is a testament to the importance of that role.

All of the above little bits of information about the thyroid gland have been crucial in fitting them together like pieces in a jigsaw puzzle to build the

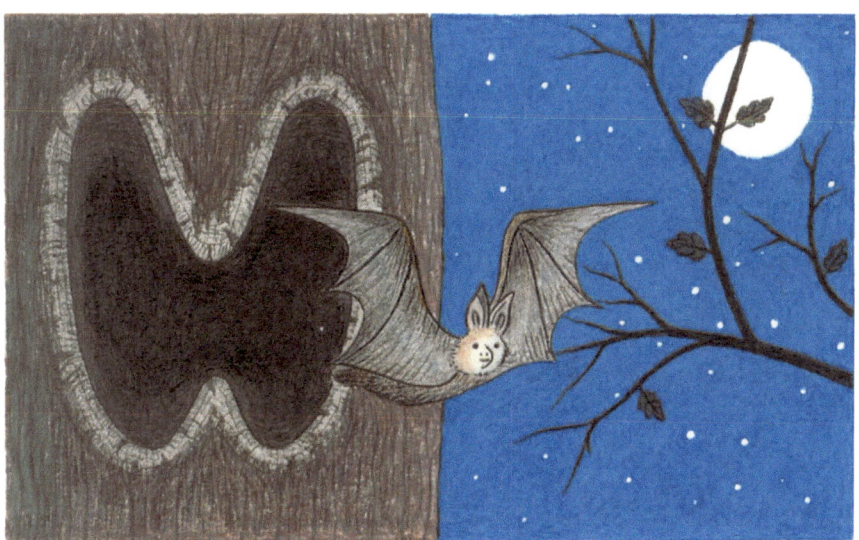

Fig. 2.6 Bats have been studied as a model for mammals that endure long periods of fasting. Profound changes in thyroid hormone levels in bats have been noted in relation to hibernation and reproductive activity [17]

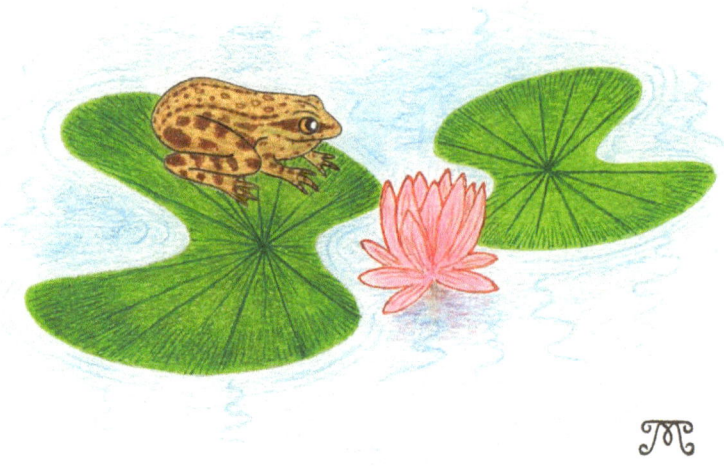

Fig. 2.7 Frogs played a role in understanding the thyroid. In 1912, experiments showed that exposing tadpoles to thyroid extract turned them to frogs [18]. For a while, tadpole metamorphosis was used to measure thyroid hormones [19]

knowledge we have today. We now know that severe iodine deficiency early in life causes cretinism not just because such children are hypothyroid but also because their brain and other tissues are not protected by the antioxidant effects of iodine.

Hypothyroidism in infancy due to causes other than iodine deficiency also interferes with mental and physical development but not to the same extent as cretinism. This is why every baby has a heel prick test shortly after being born to rule out congenital hypothyroidism. When hypothyroidism is detected in newborns and treated with thyroid hormones, growth and development (physical and mental) are unaffected.

Mild degrees of iodine deficiency cause endemic goitre, which is an adaptation of the thyroid to low levels of iodine. The thyroid grows in order to become more efficient at extracting every little bit of iodine available. When the supply of iodine to the thyroid does not meet the needs, then hypothyroidism sets in. We also know that hypothyroidism can develop in the absence of iodine deficiency as a result of 'autoimmunity'. Autoimmune hypothyroidism or otherwise known as 'Hashimoto's thyroiditis' or 'Hashimoto's disease' develops because the body's immune system attacks and destroys the thyroid gland. Hashimoto's thyroiditis is the commonest cause of hypothyroidism in iodine-sufficient parts of the world. The patients with myxoedema that Ord described in 1884 had a version of autoimmune hypothyroidism associated with shrinkage of the thyroid gland.

A Musical Night Out

The way that the human body uses thyroid hormones is complicated and not fully understood. There are numerous components that interact with each other aiming to keep the right amount of thyroid hormones delivered to different tissues and cells in the body. Here are the key players:

- The thyroid cells that form the thyroid gland and make thyroid hormones
- The 'anterior pituitary gland', the master endocrine gland of the body situated deep behind the nose at the base of the brain
- The 'thyroid stimulating hormone' (TSH) also known as 'thyrotropin' or 'thyrotrophin'). TSH is made by the anterior pituitary, which in turn controls the thyroid cells
- The hypothalamus (situated deep in the brain), which makes a hormone called 'TSH releasing hormone' (TRH) that controls the release of TSH by the anterior pituitary

Imagine that the cells in the body are the audience of a symphony and require a constant supply of good music in order to do their job well (Fig. 2.8). Think of the thyroid hormones (T4 and T3) as the music that flows and echoes around the concert hall (the human body). The levels in the bloodstream (like the notes in the score of the symphony) show small oscillations that are harmonious, but they stay in tune (within a narrow range).

The music is played by the Thyroid Philharmonic (the thyroid gland), a collection of highly skilled players (thyroid cells) that produce the music (T4 and T3). The conductor (the anterior pituitary gland) controls the orchestra (thyroid gland) through his baton (TSH). If the music needs to be played quietly, the conductor signals 'pianissimo' (low TSH); when it needs to be loud, 'fortissimo' (high TSH). It is a finely tuned dialogue between the orchestra and the conductor. The conductor is accountable to the producer (the hypothalamus), who is less visible, but highly connected and calls all the shots through messages (TRH) that are sent to the conductor (the anterior pituitary gland).

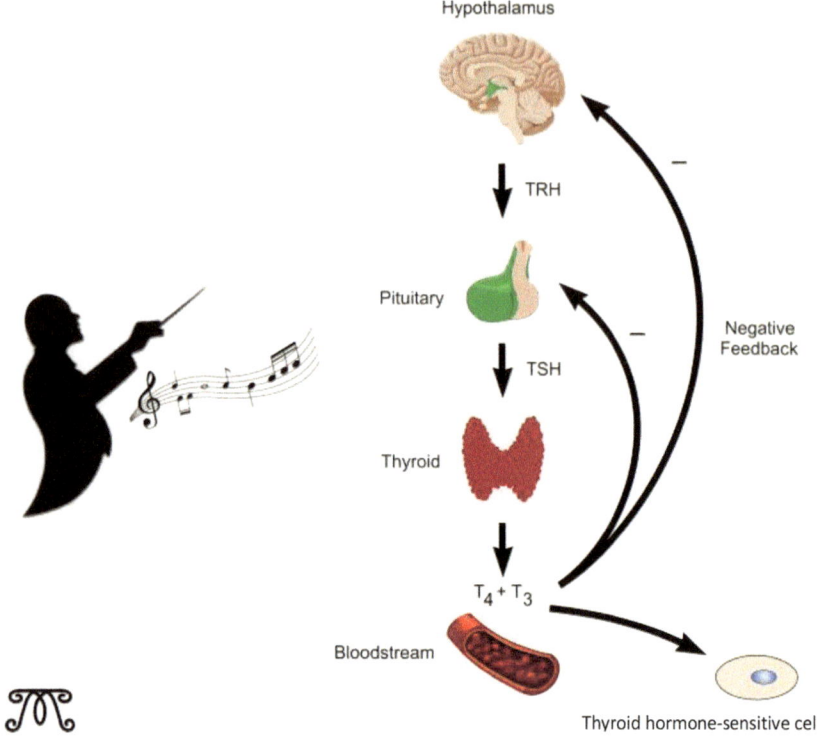

Fig. 2.8 Harmonious hormones. *TSH* thyroid-stimulating hormone, *TRH* TSH-releasing hormone, *T4* thyroxine, *T3* tri-iodothyronine, *TH* thyroid hormone

If the reader desires to delve deeper, there is a need to learn more Thyrish, and you may not feel up to it, so you can skip the next section. CoMICs is a highly recommended website with great simulations about the thyroid, and I would urge you to visit it [20].

So, the thyroid is controlled by the anterior pituitary gland through TSH, and the pituitary is controlled by the hypothalamus through TRH. In turn, the thyroid sends its messages (thyroid hormones) to other organs so that they keep doing what they are designed to do, be it the heart beating, the brain thinking or the gut digesting. Thyroid hormones also feedback on the anterior pituitary and hypothalamus reporting on the status quo, rather like a thermostat in a central heating system, so that the temperature is kept constant.

The above is an oversimplification. There are other important players that we know of and no doubt others waiting to be discovered:

- Proteins in the bloodstream that ferry thyroid hormones around
- 'Transporters' that act as revolving doors and help the passage of thyroid hormones from the fluid that bathes cells to their interior
- 'Deiodinase' enzymes that activate or neutralise thyroid hormones inside or on the surface of different cells
- Different types of 'thyroid hormone receptors' the ultimate locks that switch on and off the genes that produce all the effects of thyroid hormones (Fig. 2.9)

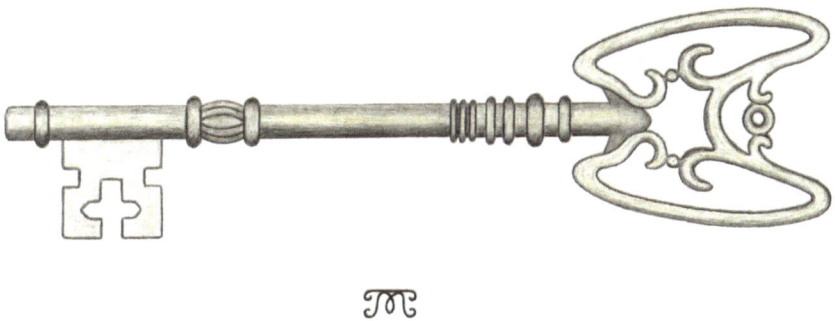

Fig. 2.9 Hormones and receptors are like keys and locks. The key has to fit precisely into the lock to switch on various functions of the cell, like making and releasing thyroid hormones

It seems that different tissues in the body (e.g. the brain or muscles) vary in their requirement of the amount of thyroid hormones, so there are local controls like transporters and deiodinases. The overall setup is a little like a central heating system in a house. You can set the overall temperature you require, but in addition, you can have smart valves on individual radiators, so you can keep your living room warmer than your bedroom and the spare room cooler than the rest of the house.

Everything about the thyroid gland is delicate, complicated, synchronised and perfectly harmonious, and the result is melodic. But it does not take much to disturb the peace and create dissonance and cacophony.

Too Little

Insufficient production of thyroid hormones leads to hypothyroidism. George Murray described the features of severe hypothyroidism (myxoedema) in great detail [21]. The commonest cause of an underactive thyroid gland globally is iodine deficiency. In regions of the world where iodine is plentiful (most developed countries) 'autoimmunity' is the commonest cause of hypothyroidism (Hashimoto's thyroiditis). Autoimmune diseases include rheumatoid arthritis, coeliac disease, multiple sclerosis, pernicious anaemia and many others. They are called autoimmune because the body's immune system turns against itself and attacks various organs causing inflammation and destruction. The attack is mounted by 'autoantibodies' (proteins made by the immune system that circulate in the bloodstream, stick to cells and tissues and may cause damage) and 'lymphocytes', which are immune cells that can also directly approach other cells and tissues and damage them.

Thyroid autoantibodies (of which there are mainly two relevant to hypothyroidism called 'thyroid peroxidase antibodies', TPOAb for short, and 'thyroglobulin antibodies') can be detected and measured in the blood and can help in making a diagnosis. Whether antibodies cause destruction of the thyroid or they are just markers of thyroid autoimmunity is unclear.

Hashimoto's thyroiditis is usually a slow process, and it takes years before its effects become apparent by producing symptoms. Part of the reason for this lies in the fact that the thyroid gland has a lot of spare capacity. In Hashimoto's thyroiditis , the thyroid gland is invaded by lymphocytes and thyroid antibodies appear in the bloodstream, but for some time, the thyroid continues to function normally, thanks to its reserve. A goitre may appear because of the large number of lymphocytes that gather there.

After a period of time (usually years), the bulk of the thyroid gland is destroyed by the immune system. At this point, the thyroid gland is unable to make enough thyroid hormones for the body's needs. As a result, the TSH level rises, and the remaining thyroid cells work harder to restore normal thyroid hormone levels. We call this 'subclinical hypothyroidism' or 'compensated hypothyroidism', characterised by raised TSH and normal thyroid hormone (T4 and T3) levels. In due course, the thyroid gland cannot keep up and fails. Then, the TSH rises further, and the T4 and T3 levels drop below normal. We call this 'overt hypothyroidism' to distinguish from 'subclinical'.

Broadly speaking, goitre associated with Hashimoto's thyroiditis tends to diminish with time and can disappear as the destruction of the thyroid progresses.

Other common causes of hypothyroidism include surgery to remove the thyroid and after treatment of an overactive thyroid with radioactive iodine.

You are likely to encounter the terms 'clinical' and 'subclinical' if you are searching for medical evidence and here is a good place to define what is meant by these terms in more detail. In everyday parlance, 'clinical' is often used to describe something that is precise, sanitary or devoid of human emotions. In medicine, 'clinical' refers to the direct interaction between a healthcare professional and a patient. So, a 'clinical' diagnosis is a diagnosis that a healthcare professional makes on the basis of the history and examination of a patient. In contrast, a diagnosis may not be evident by history and examination but may be revealed by a laboratory test and we call that 'subclinical'.

Too Much

We can get further insight into what the thyroid gland does by considering what happens when it becomes overactive and releases too much thyroid hormones into the bloodstream. Robert Graves, an eminent Irish doctor, gave a detailed description of hyperthyroidism in 1835: '*I have lately seen three cases of violent and long continued palpitations in females, in each of which the same peculiarity presented itself viz enlargement of the thyroid gland*' [22].

Later, his own name became associated with the commonest cause of hyperthyroidism, Graves' disease. Legend has it that Robert Graves invented the second hand on watches in order to measure the pulse rate of his hyperthyroid patients [23]. But it was another German doctor, Carl Adolph von Basedow, who provided the most meticulous description of autoimmune hyperthyroidism in 1840 [24] (Fig. 2.10).

Graves' disease is the commonest cause of thyroid overactivity in humans in iodine-sufficient areas. It is an autoimmune disease, but the abnormality here is that the body makes antibodies that fit into the TSH receptor on thyroid cells and switch it on. As a result, the thyroid cells receive a signal that imitates that of TSH and respond as if there is not enough thyroid hormone in the body, so they produce large amounts of T4 and T3. Because production is turned up, the thyroid gland often is enlarged in Graves' disease. The levels of T4 and T3 in the circulation are high, and TSH is low (because the high T4 and T3 levels feed back to the anterior pituitary and hypothalamus and switch off TRH and TSH production). The antibodies that stimulate the thyroid can be measured (known as 'TSH receptor antibodies' or 'TRAb'), and this is a useful diagnostic test for Graves' disease.

Other less common causes of hyperthyroidism are 'toxic multinodular goitre' and 'toxic adenomas'. These are not autoimmune (so antibody tests are typically negative) and come about as a result of groups of thyroid cells (called 'nodules') becoming more active than their neighbours and ceasing to obey the instructions of the anterior pituitary. In some cases, this seems to happen because they acquire mutations of the TSH receptor that gets stuck in the 'on' position. There are several other much rarer causes of thyroid overactivity that are beyond the scope of this book.

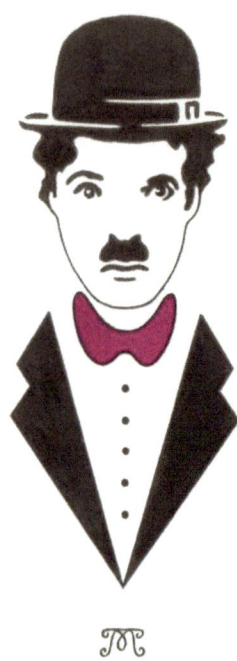

Fig. 2.10 Hyperthyroid patients are constantly on the go, a bit like Charly Chaplin. Chaplin did not have hyperthyroidism as far as is known but an unkind rival gave a graphic account of his mannerisms that implicated his thyroid: 'Chaplin squatting grey and nude, atop his chiffonier, swinging his thyroid around his head by his bamboo cane, like a dead rat' [25]

Popping Eyes

Some patients with Graves' disease develop eye problems. This is called 'thyroid eye disease', but it has many other names, just to confuse the reader (e.g. 'Graves' ophthalmopathy', 'Graves' orbitopathy', and 'endocrine exophthalmos'). Thyroid eye disease is also an autoimmune condition and causes inflammation of the tissues (muscles, fat and connective tissue) inside the socket and around the eyeball. The swelling pushes the eyeballs forward and can cause many distressing symptoms [26].

Thyroid Lumps

Thyroid lumps are common. Up to about 5% of adults have a thyroid lump that can be seen or felt with our fingers. Using a sensitive imaging technique like ultrasound, small thyroid lumps can be found in more than 50% of adults. A single thyroid lump or multiple discrete lumps are referred to as a 'nodule' or 'nodules'. When multiple lumps make the thyroid gland overall enlarged, it is referred to as 'multinodular goitre'. But these are just descriptive terms and say nothing about the nature of the lumps.

Thyroid nodules can be 'benign' (innocent) or 'malignant' (cancerous). The vast majority of thyroid lumps are benign. When a thyroid lump appears, it needs to be diagnosed as either benign or malignant. An ultrasound of the thyroid is a useful test, and it can confidently identify most benign and some malignant nodules. However, a sizeable proportion of thyroid nodules (about 30%) have an 'indeterminate' appearance on ultrasound, and such cases usually are referred for a needle biopsy. In many cases, the needle biopsy settles the question, but in some, it does not help and the nodule needs to be removed surgically for a definitive diagnosis.

Summing It All Up

From the first description of the thyroid gland as an organ in the sixteenth century to the discovery of the treatment of hypothyroidism with sheep thyroid extract in 1891, knowledge about the thyroid was largely based on observations that often resulted in misleading interpretations. From the twentieth century onwards, scientific investigations were enriched by new technologies, which increasingly made more accurate measurements of chemical substances in the body. This led to an explosion of experimental studies that involved human beings, animals and cells in test tubes. The new knowledge provided novel explanations and understanding of the way the thyroid gland functions and the causes of thyroid diseases. As a result, new treatments were developed. Doctors had to absorb all the new knowledge and translate it into medical practice.

The next chapter explores evidence-based medicine, how scientific studies are reported in the medical literature and how different studies are classified.

References

1. Vaccarella S, Franceschi S, Bray F, Wild CP, Plummer M, Dal Maso L. Worldwide thyroid-cancer epidemic? The increasing impact of overdiagnosis. N Engl J Med. 2016;375(7):614–7. https://doi.org/10.1056/NEJMp1604412.
2. Durante C, Grani G, Lamartina L, Filetti S, Mandel SJ, Cooper DS. The diagnosis and management of thyroid nodules: a review. JAMA. 2018;319(9):914–24. https://doi.org/10.1001/jama.2018.0898.

 3. Lydiatt DD, Bucher GS. Historical vignettes of the thyroid gland. Clin Anat. 2011;24(1):1–9. https://doi.org/10.1002/ca.21073.
 4. Wharton T. Adenographia: sive glandularum totius corporis descriptio. Amstelaedami: Sumptibus Joannis Ravesteinii; 1659.
 5. Lazzeri D, Pozzilli P. "Madonna of the carnation": Leonardo da Vinci (1452-1519). J Endocrinol Invest. 2018;41(7):879–80. https://doi.org/10.1007/s40618-018-0842-z.
 6. Rush B. An inquiry into the functions of the spleen, liver, pancreas, and thyroid gland. Med Phys J. 1806;16(91):193–208.
 7. Wesche MF, Wiersinga WM, Smits NJ. Lean body mass as a determinant of thyroid size. Clin Endocrinol (Oxf). 1998;48(6):701–6. https://doi.org/10.1046/j.1365-2265.1998.00400.x.
 8. Slater S. The discovery of thyroid replacement therapy. Part 1: in the beginning. J R Soc Med. 2011;104(1):15–8. https://doi.org/10.1258/jrsm.2010.10k050.
 9. Merke F. History and iconography of endemic goitre and cretinism. MTP Press; 1984.
10. Ord W. Clinical lecture on myxoedema. Br Med J. 1878;1(906):671–2.
11. Rosenfeld L. Discovery and early uses of iodine. J Chem Educ. 2000;77(8):984–7. https://doi.org/10.1021/ed077p984.
12. Murray GR. Note on the treatment of myxoedema by hypodermic injections of an extract of the thyroid gland of a sheep. Br Med J. 1891;2(1606):796–7. https://doi.org/10.1136/bmj.2.1606.796.
13. Kohrle J, Biebermann H. 3-iodothyronamine-A thyroid hormone metabolite with distinct target profiles and mode of action. Endocr Rev. 2019;40(2):602–30. https://doi.org/10.1210/er.2018-00182.
14. Venturi S, Venturi M. Evolution of dietary antioxidant defences. Eur EPI-Marker. 2007;11(3):1–12.
15. Kupper FC, Carpenter LJ, McFiggans GB, et al. Iodide accumulation provides kelp with an inorganic antioxidant impacting atmospheric chemistry. Proc Natl Acad Sci U S A. 2008;105(19):6954–8. https://doi.org/10.1073/pnas.0709959105.
16. Heyland A, Moroz LL. Cross-kingdom hormonal signaling: an insight from thyroid hormone functions in marine larvae. J Exp Biol. 2005;208(Pt 23):4355–61. https://doi.org/10.1242/jeb.01877.
17. Martinez B, Ortiz RM. Thyroid hormone regulation and insulin resistance: insights from animals naturally adapted to fasting. Physiology (Bethesda). 2017;32(2):141–51. https://doi.org/10.1152/physiol.00018.2016.
18. Gudernatsch JF. Feeding experiments on tadpoles: I. The influence of specific organs given as food on growth and differentiation. A contribution to the knowledge of organs with internal secretion. Wilhelm Roux Arch Entwicklungsmech Organismen. 1912;35:457–83.
19. Gaddum JH. Quantitative observations on thyroxine and allied substances: I. The use of tadpoles. J Physiol. 1927–1928;64:246.

20. CoMICs. https://sites.google.com/view/simbasimulation/comics/comics-lite?authuser=0.
21. Murray GR. Diseases of the thyroid gland. H.K. Lewis; 1900.
22. Graves R. https://archive.org/details/p2londonmedicals07londuoft/page/516/mode/2up/search/thyroid.
23. Williams DL. A history of graves and St. John's. Eye (Lond). 2019;33(2):174–5. https://doi.org/10.1038/s41433-018-0267-0.
24. Basedow CA. Exophthalmus durch Hypertrophie des Zellgewebes in der Augenhoehle. Wochenschrift fuer die Gesamte Heilkunde. 1840;13:197–204.
25. CharlieChaplin. http://adrinkershistoryoflondon.com/tag/charlie-chaplin/.
26. Perros P, Krassas GE. Graves orbitopathy: a perspective. Nat Rev Endocrinol. 2009;5(6):312–8. https://doi.org/10.1038/nrendo.2009.61.

3

What Is the Evidence?

'The most convincing argument that evidence-based medicine is a positive development in healthcare, is the dramatic improvement in survival of children with cancer'

Taking the Stand

'What is the evidence?' is a question that thyroid patients, carers and the lay public often ask their doctor. Doctors also ask themselves the same question before making important decisions. Other interested stakeholders include pharmacists, managers, regulators and funders of healthcare. Trying to answer this question can feel like being interrogated by the prosecutor in a court. The stakes are high, and the consequences of the answer can be serious.

Besides thinking about what constitutes evidence, it is important to have some idea of how evidence is generated, disseminated and applied and the ups and downs that go with it. Awareness of these bedfellows of medical evidence and the processes at work that are involved in turning observations and experimentation into medical evidence will help the quest for truth.

In this chapter, you will find the basics about evidence-based medicine and how it translates to practice. But first, let me introduce you to Peggy.

© The Author(s), under exclusive license to Springer Nature Switzerland AG 2024
P. Perros, *Seeking Thyroid Truths*, Copernicus Books,
https://doi.org/10.1007/978-3-031-58287-5_3

Peggy's Hedgehogs

Peggy, an 83-year old pateint, sat uncomfortably in my consulting room next to her daughter. Peggy did not wish to speak. In fact her body language screamed that she would rather give birth to twin hedgehogs than be in my clinic that morning. So, most of the talking was done by her daughter.

The story in short was that Peggy was getting frail and 'losing her marbles'. The family doctor had done some investigations and found that her thyroid blood tests were marginally abnormal, something we call in Thyrish 'subclinical hyperthyroidism'. Subclinical hyperthyroidism is borderline thyroid over-activity, which usually is insufficient to cause symptoms. The daughter had 'done her research' and come to the conclusion that subclinical hyperthyroidism caused her mom's dementia. There are some evidence-based recommendations in favour of treating subclinical hyperthyroidism under specific circumstances (dementia is not among them) [1], and it would have been dead easy to send mother and daughter off with a prescription. However, while the association between subclinical hyperthyroidism and dementia is not in doubt, studies of patients with subclinical hyperthyroidism who have been treated are unconvincing about benefits (except when there is a rapid and irregular heart beat called 'atrial fibrillation'), and the treatments for subclinical hyperthyroidism carry risks [1]. In other words (remember the rooster's crow, which makes the sun rise in Chap. 1?), the daughter's argument was not that far off, suggesting that by turning the bird into coq au vin, we could make the night last forever.

I was clear in my mind that the extremely unlikely possibility that Peggy's forgetfulness would improve with treatment was outweighed by the risks and hassles of treatment. For instance, treatment could potentially make her hypothyroid and exacerbate her existing problems and cause side effects, and she would need regular blood tests and adjustments in her medication.

After a lengthy discussion and eventual engagement from Peggy, it became apparent that although she was in the early stages of dementia, she was able to understand what this was about, including the consequences of having treatment or no treatment. She made it clear that she did not wish to be treated and eventually left my consulting room without a prescription, with everyone satisfied (including the daughter) that this was the right decision for Peggy.

Peggy's story highlights that after considering the medical evidence, the final act of decision-making between patient and doctor is a process that includes sharing relevant information in a manner that the patient can understand. It requires participation by both parties in decision-making. The doctor should take into account the individual circumstances of the patient, their values, choices and ultimately respect their autonomy. This principle is also one of the pillars of medical ethics.

Doctors occasionally act against evidence-based guidelines and recommendations, because it is the right thing to do for that particular patient. One point worth mentioning is that although a patient can refuse a treatment that a doctor proposes, a doctor has the right (indeed is ethically obliged) to refuse a treatment that a patient may wish to have if the doctor judges that on balance that treatment is likely harmful for that patient. This can cause a great deal of conflict, resentment and dissatisfaction as patients may feel that they themselves are the best judges of what is good for them. There are no easy solutions to this, as we have seen in the case of the controversy that surrounds liothyronine treatment for hypothyroidism. One sure lesson is that appeals to politicians to intervene and adjudicate are futile [2]. The answer in such cases lies in engaging doctors and patients in dialogue, guided by the impartial interpretation of the evidence, negotiating and, if necessary, seeking a second opinion.

Evidence-Based Medicine

Evidence-based medicine is the cornerstone of modern medical practice. It emerged as an antidote to the failures of a previous era when numerous treatments, now proven to be ineffective or even harmful, were being widely used. Drilling holes in the skull ('trepanation') or surgical removal of part of the brain ('lobotomy') for mental illness, use of mercury (a highly toxic chemical) for syphilis, and radium as an elixir for various ailments are just some such examples. Bloodletting was practiced for over 2000 years and was based on the belief that illness was due to an imbalance in the 'humours' of the body. Some of these gruesome remedies were not abandoned in some places until the twentieth century.

It now seems remarkable that such 'treatments' flourished for so long, but the capacity of the human body to rid itself of many common ailments and the 'placebo' effect can probably account for that ('placebo' is a psychologically beneficial effect of a medication or procedure that in reality has no healing effect).

Nowadays, the entire institutions are dedicated to appraising and implementing evidence-based medicine, like the National Institute for Health and Care Excellence (NICE), the Cochrane database for systematic reviews, the

Centre for Evidence-based medicine in Oxford and the Institute for Clinical and Economic Review in the USA.

Evidence builds up from observations and experimentation in test tubes, on animals, or humans. The information is collected and analysed, and the knowledge is turned into 'hypotheses' or theories that are probable explanations for what is being observed. Whenever possible, the observations should be repeated and verified. Observations that are not reproducible are unlikely to represent true events. Hypotheses are tested and based on the results are rejected, modified and retested. The cycle repeats itself in perpetuity, and with every round, we learn more and get closer to the truth.

Evidence is based as much as possible on objective assessments, hence the obsession of science with measurements. It is also based on rational thinking. Sentiments, emotions and gut feelings have no place in generating medical evidence.

Spreading the News

Medical evidence is spread across the medical and scientific community mainly through publications in academic journals. Findings from medical research reach their readers in small bites. Each one makes up an entity, but is a tiny part of the bigger picture. Do not expect a single publication of original research to provide the answer to a big question. Breakthroughs happen rarely. The vast majority of the findings of medical research is published in journals rather than books. This reflects the enormous new information that is generated from research every day, which putting into books would be a big task and would run the risk of being outdated by the time the book is published.

The Publication Process

Being 'published' is a big deal, but not all publications are equal. If you wish to improve your ability to appraise the evidence, then it will help to have some understanding of how pieces of evidence are selected for publication.

Once authors are satisfied that their material merits publication, they will start to think about choosing a suitable journal. Some medical journals specialise in particular types of study. For example, studies on humans, or animals, or purely laboratory-based experiments (referred to as 'basic' research), while others concentrate on turning the knowledge from basic research into treatments ('translational' research). Some journals will accept any kind of medical specialty (e.g. the *New England Journal of Medicine, Lancet, Journal of the American Medical Association* and *British Medical Journal*). Others are oriented towards a specialty like endocrinology (e.g. *Journal of Clinical Endocrinology and Metabolism, European Journal of Endocrinology* and *Clinical Endocrinology*) or a subspecialty (e.g. *European Thyroid Journal, Thyroid* and *Thyroid Research*).

Impact Factor

Besides choosing a journal that best fits the subject of a paper, authors are also mindful of the journal 'impact factor'. Impact factor is a popular quality metric for a journal [3]. It is a number derived from the number of times publications in that journal are cited by other publications. It assumes that ground-breaking publications are cited frequently, while unimportant research is rarely mentioned by other researchers.

It is common for authors to start with a high-impact factor journal and if rejected to step downwards. The highest impact factor in 2021 was 176 held by the *New England Journal of Medicine* [4]. The impact factors of some popular endocrine/thyroid journals are shown below.

Journal	Impact factor	Year
Nature Reviews Endocrinology	47.6 (Nature portfolio)	2021
Endocrine Reviews	25.3	2021
Thyroid	6.5	2021
Journal of Clinical Endocrinology and Metabolism	6.1	2021
Journal of Endocrinological Investigation	5.5	2021
European Thyroid Journal	4.1	'Latest'
Clinical Endocrinology	3.4	2019
Hormone and Metabolic Research	2.2	2022
Thyroid Research		Not available
Journal of Thyroid Research		Not available

Peer Review

Once the paper is received by the journal, the 'peer-review' process begins. The editor usually decides if the topic is appropriate or not for that particular journal, and if so, whether the findings are of sufficient quality and interest to merit consideration. If not, the paper is rejected; otherwise, it enters the next phase during which two to four (occasionally one or more than four) peer reviewers assess the paper independently. Some journals have teams of statisticians who also scrutinise the numbers and statistical methods used.

Peer reviewers are academic experts in the field. It is exceptional for a paper to be accepted without requiring some form of revision. Most submissions are rejected. Rejection rates vary from 40 to 90% or more, which is another metric of journal quality. The remainder are required to undergo minor or major revisions based on the peer reviewers' comments. Authors are provided with written critiques and may be invited to submit their revised paper. Ultimately, the editor decides to accept or reject a paper, but it would be very unusual for the editor's decision to be radically different to that of the peer reviewers.

Peer review is an important part of the publication process and safeguards a minimum standard of quality, in the same way that it is reassuring to know that an obscure airline whose aircraft you are about to board is certified by the International Air Transport Association. Conversely, medical evidence that is not peer reviewed should raise concerns about its validity.

Peer reviewers are not paid for their services as this activity is regarded as one that an academic is expected to deliver. Many journals apply article publication charges payable by the authors or their academic institutions and fees for making the full text of the paper available to the public, which can vary from under $100 to €9500 [5]. These financial impositions are sometimes barriers to disseminating scientific knowledge.

Architecture of Medical Papers

Most papers have a common structure. First come the authors and the title of the paper. The number of authors can range from 1 to over 1000 (though usually not more than half a dozen). This reflects the complexity of medical research and the collaborative nature of this activity.

Following the author list is the abstract, which is a brief summary. Abstracts of papers are nearly always available online, so they are accessible to everyone. The main text is usually divided into an introduction, which provides the background and context of the study and outlines the objectives. It is followed by a description of the methods used, then comes the results section. In the discussion section, the results are interpreted, and one or more conclusions are drawn.

The final section is the list of references. In addition, there are usually figures and tables, and there may be additional supplementary information. The paper may also include a description of the contribution of each co-author, potential conflicts of interest, funding sources and acknowledgements.

Keywords are usually mentioned at the beginning of papers. They are used for indexing purposes and identify the most important items covered by the paper. The results of searches that you have done were probably generated by matching your keywords with those of published papers.

Types of Medical Evidence

There are several types of medical research and publications that can be classified in various ways. The classification I have chosen is commonly used and one I prefer (Fig. 3.1). Before diving into the specific types of published evidence, it is worth highlighting the distinction between 'primary' (or original) and 'secondary' sources of evidence.

Primary papers present data from studies that have not been published previously. 'Secondary' are papers about primary publications. They can be opinion pieces (commentaries, editorials, letters to the editor), narrative reviews, systematic reviews, meta-analyses, guidelines or consensus statements (described in more detail below).

Primary evidence may be 'observational', reporting on something interesting or unusual that happens. In contrast, 'interventional' studies usually

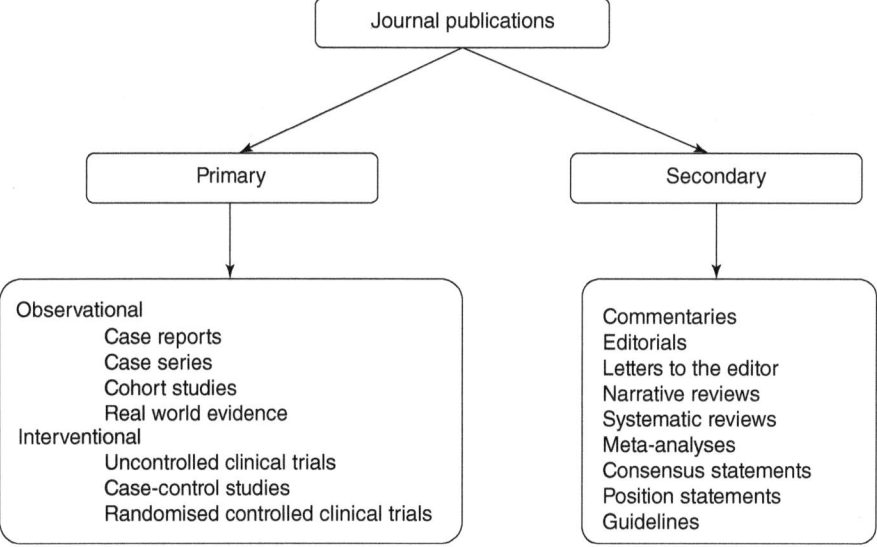

Fig. 3.1 Types of journal publications

involve a treatment (the intervention) and an assessment of its outcome. Primary evidence can be 'retrospective' (looking at past records) or 'prospective' (starting at a certain point in time at the beginning of the study and recording what happens after a set time period). Some studies are 'cross-sectional' (they describe something that is observed at one single time, like a snapshots), others are 'longitudinal' (they follow patients up for a period of time). Longitudinal studies can be about a group of patients who have already been followed up for a period of time and data can be extracted from their records retrospectively, or the study can commence after the protocol has been agreed and the data are collected prospectively. Cross-sectional designs are appropriate for some types of research questions, for example, for working out if a diagnostic test is better than another, but not for others (e.g. studying the causes of a disease). So, the study design to a large extent is dependent on what the research question is, for example, what is the cause of a disease?, how to diagnose it?, what is the long-term outlook? and how effective is a treatment?

Primary Evidence

Case Reports

Case reports are descriptions of something related to a patient that is unusual and insightful. Most case reports are of limited value, but there are exceptions. For instance, George Murray's first description of a patient being treated with sheep thyroid extract for myxoedema in 1891 [6]. Murray's case report can be described as 'prospective' (it was planned in advance), 'interventional' (it involved administering a treatment) and 'longitudinal' (he recorded the features of hypothyroidism before and sometime after treatment). Case reports can be informative especially when they are about rare diseases or rare but serious side effects of treatments, but most are of very limited value, so they are usually placed at the bottom of the pile for quality.

Case Series

Case series are similar to case reports but contain a larger numbers of patients, usually from the same centre. Case series are descriptive and limited in scientific content, usually retrospective and subject to bias. However, for rare diseases, they may be the only source of information available. An example was a collection of 13 patients with 'Hashimoto's encephalopathy' (a very rare but serious brain condition associated with Hashimoto's thyroiditis) from a single Chinese centre collected over 5 years [7]. It showed that patients treated with steroids had a better outlook (so the study was prospective, interventional and longitudinal). The small numbers of patients rendered the findings inconclusive but of some interest.

Cohort Studies

Cohort studies take us further up the respectability scale of medical research (Fig. 3.2) and because of the larger numbers of patients than case series, they are able to compensate for some of the bias. Cohort studies focus on populations with some common characteristic (e.g. patients with a diagnosis of hypothyroidism) and record data at baseline and some subsequent interval(s). Such a cohort study showed that a slightly raised serum TSH (subclinical hypothyroidism) is a normal finding in old people and it was associated with living longer than people with a normal TSH [8] (the study was prospective, observational and longitudinal). This was clearly an important finding, which impacts on decision-making about the treatment.

One reason why cohort studies are the right design for some types of research, for instance, if one wishes to work out the outlook of patients with a diagnosis of thyroid cancer.

One particular type of case series/cohort studies on a massive scale is 'real-world evidence' (RWE) [9], which has been made possible by 'big data' that are collected digitally. RWE is gathered from electronic health records of

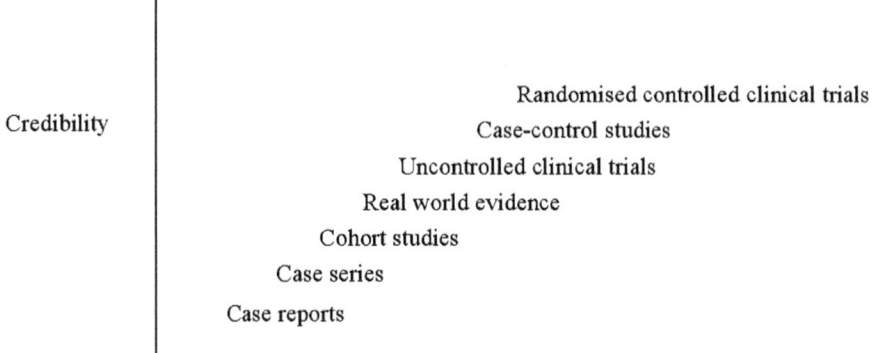

ORIGINAL STUDIES

Credibility

Randomised controlled clinical trials
Case-control studies
Uncontrolled clinical trials
Real world evidence
Cohort studies
Case series
Case reports

Fig. 3.2 Simplified overview of scientific value of studies by study design

populations, claims and billing data, product and disease registries, and data gathered through personal devices and health applications, which can be very large in numbers [10]. This approach is easier, less expensive and quicker than other types of study, but potential traps and flaws also abound. The quality of the data that RWE studies are based on may be not as good as those collected by teams of researchers, and the methods used to analyse the data can sometimes be misleading. Nonetheless, RWE is proliferating at a great rate and is already contributing significantly to our knowledge of thyroid-related topics [11–13].

Uncontrolled Clinical Trials

Uncontrolled clinical trials (we call them 'uncontrolled' because they lack a comparative or 'control' group) look at the effect of a treatment by measuring an outcome before and after treatment. Note that the word 'trial' is used in medical research to describe a study that involves a treatment (drug or device or procedure). Uncontrolled trials can be misleading because many human diseases and symptoms improve spontaneously or as a result of the placebo effect. A particularly bad example of an uncontrolled trial was by Luzina et al. [14], both in terms of study design and execution. The authors assessed the effects of acupuncture on subclinical hypothyroidism. It was a poorly designed study (small number of patients, inadequate description of how they were selected and absence of a control group), thus casting serious doubts on the validity of the conclusions that acupuncture was an effective treatment (unsurprisingly the study was published in an obscure journal with an impact factor of 0.35). However, uncontrolled clinical trials may be the only way of investigating some treatments and can provide valuable data. Phase I and phase II clinical trials are uncontrolled and look at the safety (phase I) and effectiveness (phase II) of new drugs without control groups and are necessary preludes to definitive evaluations (phase III) of treatments.

Case-Control Studies

Case-control studies look at whether a group defined by a diagnosis or exposure to the treatment or a risk factor has an outcome that is different to a comparative control group; however, the control group has not entered the study at the same time or with the same criteria as the cases (subjects) that are being studied. Case-control studies can be observational or interventional. It is the study design of choice when exploring whether something potentially harmful (e.g. chemicals in the environment) can cause the disease. It is not the design of choice when testing the effects of a treatment as bias creeps in, and the results are not easy to interpret.

An example of an interventional case-control study was one that examined whether 'near-total thyroidectomy' (an operation to remove most of the thyroid gland) had a more beneficial effect on the outcome of thyroid eye disease than the treatment with anti-thyroid drugs [15]. A group of patients with Graves' disease, some of whom had thyroid eye disease was treated with 'near-total thyroidectomy' (almost complete removal of the thyroid gland by surgery). The outcomes with regard to the thyroid eye disease 12 months post-operatively were compared with the records of a group of patients with Graves' disease who had been treated in the same hospital with anti-thyroid drugs. No differences were found between the two groups. Although the control subjects were matched for age, sex, duration of hyperthyroidism and severity of thyroid eye disease, other differences may well have influenced the results. The group treated with surgery, for instance, may have included more patients with large goitres or patients suspected of having thyroid cancer (these characteristics make it more likely that surgery is chosen than drugs). Also since the two groups were not studied at the same time, the doctors who performed the examination of the eyes may have been different in the two groups of patients and the way they assessed and recorded their findings may have varied.

Randomised Controlled Clinical Trials

In 'randomised controlled clinical trials', treatments are allocated to groups of patients at random (which takes away some of the bias). If the subjects and the investigators are aware who received which treatment before the study is completed, they are referred to as 'non-blinded'. This is important as knowledge by either patients or researchers of what treatment is being used can affect the outcomes of such studies and should be interpreted with care.

The king of medical research for assessing interventions is the randomised 'double-blinded' controlled clinical trial also known as 'phase III trial'. Neither patient nor researcher knows which treatment corresponds to which patient (hence, 'double-blinded'), until the study is complete.

Here is an example of a randomised controlled study in a topic that is of interest to patients with hypothyroidism. 'Fine tuning' the levothyroxine dose is often discussed, and there are strong opinions on this based on individual patient experiences. Samuels et al. [16] did a large double-blinded, randomised controlled trial, which contrary to popular thinking, showed no differences in quality of life, mood or cognition in patients achieving levels of TSH ranging from low to high (0.34–12 mU/L).

Secondary Evidence

Commentaries, Editorials and Letters to the Editor

Commentaries are usually commissioned by the journal to an expert who puts forward his/her opinion on a paper that is published in the same issue of the journal. Commentaries are published because the original piece of research that they discuss is of particular interest. Editorials are similar to commentaries but are written by one of the editors and represent the journal opinion and carry more weight than commentaries. Letters to the editor are written by any reader of the journal who wishes to share a view. Commentaries, editorials and letters to the editor are largely personal opinions, though they may provide interesting perspectives and stimulate new ideas.

Narrative Reviews, Systematic Reviews and Meta-analyses

Narrative reviews, systematic reviews and meta-analyses aim to evaluate previously published original research on a theme or topic. 'Narrative reviews' tell a story about a subject and original research that the authors consider relevant, upon which their interpretations and opinions are formulated and expressed. 'Systematic reviews' also focus on a specific topic or question and consider all the relevant evidence, but unlike narrative reviews, they use clearly defined methods for selecting the relevant evidence. 'Meta-analyses' use valid statistical methods to combine the results from several similar studies.

Guidelines and Consensus Statements

Guidelines use all the available evidence, including systematic reviews and meta-analyses, to formulate recommendations on how patients should be managed in real life. Guidelines are produced by panels of experts who evaluate all the evidence and reach consensus on investigations and treatments, which are intended to support doctors in their daily practice. Guidelines are a way of condensing a large amount of knowledge into a set of rules that are likely to lead to desirable results.

Imagine having to drive from one end of a foreign city to another, a city that you have never visited before, let alone drive in, and it is rush hour. Oh, by the way, it's in Italy, so you are surrounded by native drivers who approach motoring as a gladiatorial pursuit by delinquent adolescents on a sugar rush. Boy, aren't you glad you have satnav! At every junction, the reassuring, yet irritating voice with the weird accent, tells you that on the grounds of probability going straight, or taking a left or right turn will get you a little closer to your destination. That's guidelines.

Consensus statements are similar to guidelines, but they tend to cover areas in medicine where the evidence is scarce, and therefore, recommendations are based more on experience and expert opinion than robust evidence.

If you are seeking an answer in guidelines and consensus statements, they will probably get you there, but don't be hugely surprised if there are unexpected hurdles on the way, for example a protest by Napolitan municipal workers or a political rally that even satnav cannot predict. Most importantly, you should not follow Miss Weird Accent blindly. If she is telling you to drive head on to a wall, you should use your own judgment and common sense, while showering her and her satnav with epithets that are best not repeated here. That does not happen with guidelines often, but it is not unheard of.

Guidelines are the distillation of medical evidence. How doctors apply them to the singular person who needs their help is the art of medicine. It comes with experience and with getting to know that person. Unfortunately, this cannot be done in a five-minute consultation. So, shortcuts are often taken, the guidelines are followed to the letter and to be fair, the result in the vast majority of cases is fine, but the patient may be left perplexed and unsatisfied with the experience. No easy answers, but let us not dismiss guidelines and evidence-based medicine because they are sometimes used inappropriately.

The Dark Side of Medical Evidence

Evidence-based medicine has its downsides and has been criticised. In 2014, the editor of the *British Medical Journal* summarised the concerns raised [17] and quoted one critic who stated that *'evidence based medicine was broken, the research pond was polluted by fraud, sham diagnosis, short term data, poor regulation, surrogate endpoints, and clinically irrelevant outcomes, and left no room for discretion and fuelled overdiagnosis and overtreatment'*. The editorial concluded that '*evidence based medicine may be the worst system for clinical decision making, except for all those other systems that have been tried from time to time. It is only as good as the evidence and the people making the decisions*'.

Some thyroid patient advocates, and some endocrinologists challenge the wisdom of recommendations developed on the principles of evidence-based medicine as applied to treating thyroid diseases, but the wisdom of the BMJ editor's conclusion should not be forgotten.

Moving on to another dark spot, published papers are sometimes retracted for a variety of reasons ranging from genuine errors to fraud. When such problems are identified, there is an investigation led by the journal where the paper was published, which may lead to a retraction. The number of retracted papers generally, including on thyroid topics, is increasing. In the last 6 months of 2022, 18 thyroid papers were retracted according to PubMed. 'Fake paper factories' are a concerning problem that seem largely to originate from certain countries [18].

Another troublesome recent trend is sales of authorship for publications [19]. Fake data publications have been facilitated by some journals with low-quality standards that fail to scrutinise the material submitted for publication and are money-making scams [20]. These are known as 'predatory journals', and their publications have burgeoned from 53,000 articles in 2010 to 420,000 in 2014 [21]. To expose predatory journals, fake data were submitted and shown that they were accepted without difficulty [22]. Jeffry Beall, a librarian, produced a list of predatory journals in his blog, which he was subsequently forced to shut down due to threats of litigation by publishers [23, 24]. Cabell's Blacklist [25] provides an alternative list of predatory journals to Beall's list; however, there are some doubts about its validity [23] and its services are not free of charge. There are other catalogues of predatory journals that a Google search will identify, but their reliability is unclear.

It is important to highlight two important remaining dark facts about the published medical literature. Firstly, studies with positive results are more likely to be published than those with negative ones, even though negatives can be just as important [26]. Secondly, studies that are funded by the pharmaceutical industry (especially when co-authors are employees) are more likely to be biased than studies funded from public sources [27].

The shady spots in academia mentioned above paint a grim picture. But the vast majority of medical publications are authored by hardworking decent people who are trying to push the boundaries of knowledge.

Why Evidence-Based Medicine Should Be Trusted?

In the thyroid field, the principles of evidence-based medicine were crucial for some of the most spectacular advances.

- The near eradication of cretinism
- The development of effective targeted treatments for some of the worst outlook thyroid cancers [28]
- The introduction of a highly effective treatment for thyroid eye disease [29]
- The introduction of minimally invasive treatments for thyroid nodules [30]
- The introduction of highly sensitive molecular tests for diagnosing thyroid tumours [31]

The most convincing argument that evidence-based medicine is a positive development in healthcare is the dramatic improvement in the survival of children with cancer, which would not have happened without the implementation of treatments based on evidence (Fig. 3.3) and, more recently, the enormous benefits of vaccine technology.

Implementation of evidence-based medicine has helped to reduce unnecessary and potentially harmful investigations, diagnose diseases (like breast and

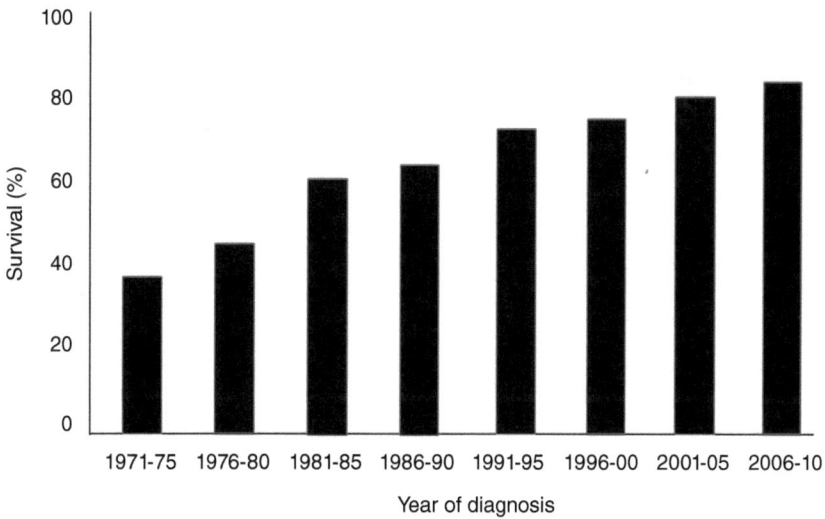

Fig. 3.3 Childhood cancer survival 1971–2010 in the UK (redrawn from Cancer Research UK) [32]

cervical cancer) early, speed up recovery post-operatively and reduce the harmful effects of smoking [33]. Highly critical views about evidence-based medicine have their roots in examples where poor science and fraud have joined forces and masqueraded as evidence-based medicine.

Some of the bad press that evidence-based medicine gets is driven by the misconception that the transition from evidence-based conclusions to dispensing treatments is merely based on following a set of rules. This could be so if human beings were identical automaton clones. In real life, the decision-making process is a fragile bridge that needs to be carefully negotiated through the interaction between physician and patient. This is why I think (and hope) that healthcare professionals will never be replaced by robots and artificial intelligence.

Take-Home Message

Now you know what evidence-based medicine is, how it is classified and how it reaches the medical literature, you are better equipped to locate and appreciate what you are looking for.

Show respect for peer-reviewed evidence published in high-impact-factor journals and for studies that are well designed for that purpose, especially randomised controlled trials. Take evidence that is not peer-reviewed with a large pinch of salt. Maintain healthy scepticism for evidence that is published in low-impact-factor journals especially case reports and retrospective series, especially if funded and authored by commercial organisations. And remember the transition from evidence-based recommendations to a decision about an individual patient is not a mathematical equation.

References

1. Biondi B, Bartalena L, Cooper DS, Hegedus L, Laurberg P, Kahaly GJ. The 2015 European Thyroid Association guidelines on diagnosis and treatment of endogenous subclinical hyperthyroidism. Eur Thyroid J. 2015;4(3):149–63. https://doi.org/10.1159/000438750.
2. ScottishParliament. http://external.parliament.scot/S5_PublicPetitionsCommittee/Reports/20180327_PE1463_thyroid.pdf.
3. Garfield E. The history and meaning of the journal impact factor. JAMA. 2006;295(1):90–3. https://doi.org/10.1001/jama.295.1.90.
4. NEJMImpactFactor. https://www.nejm.org/about-nejm/about-nejm.

5. ArticlePublicationCharges. https://en.wikipedia.org/wiki/Article_processing_charge.

6. Murray GR. Note on the treatment of myxoedema by hypodermic injections of an extract of the thyroid gland of a sheep. Br Med J. 1891;2(1606):796–7. https://doi.org/10.1136/bmj.2.1606.796.

7. Tang Y, Xing Y, Lin MT, Zhang J, Jia J. Hashimoto's encephalopathy cases: Chinese experience. BMC Neurol. 2012;12:60. https://doi.org/10.1186/1471-2377-12-60.

8. Gussekloo J, van Exel E, de Craen AJ, Meinders AE, Frolich M, Westendorp RG. Thyroid status, disability and cognitive function, and survival in old age. JAMA. 2004;292(21):2591–9. https://doi.org/10.1001/jama.292.21.2591.

9. Okun S. The missing reality of real life in real-world evidence. Clin Pharmacol Ther. 2019;106(1):136–8. https://doi.org/10.1002/cpt.1465.

10. Sherman RE, Anderson SA, Dal Pan GJ, et al. Real-world evidence—what is it and what can it tell us? N Engl J Med. 2016;375(23):2293–7. https://doi.org/10.1056/NEJMsb1609216.

11. Abrahamsen B, Jorgensen HL, Laulund AS, et al. The excess risk of major osteoporotic fractures in hypothyroidism is driven by cumulative hyperthyroid as opposed to hypothyroid time: an observational register-based time-resolved cohort analysis. J Bone Miner Res. 2015;30(5):898–905. https://doi.org/10.1002/jbmr.2416.

12. Hepp Z, Lage MJ, Espaillat R, Gossain VV. The association between adherence to levothyroxine and economic and clinical outcomes in patients with hypothyroidism in the US. J Med Econ. 2018;21(9):912–9. https://doi.org/10.1080/13696998.2018.1484749.

13. Thayakaran R, Adderley NJ, Sainsbury C, et al. Thyroid replacement therapy, thyroid stimulating hormone concentrations, and long term health outcomes in patients with hypothyroidism: longitudinal study. BMJ. 2019;366:l4892. https://doi.org/10.1136/bmj.l4892.

14. Luzina KE, Luzina LL, Vasilenko AM. [The influence of acupuncture on the quality of life and the level of thyroid-stimulating hormone in patients presenting with subclinical hypothyroidism]. Vopr Kurortol Fizioter Lech Fiz Kult. 2011;(5):29–33.

15. Marcocci C, Bruno-Bossio G, Manetti L, et al. The course of Graves' ophthalmopathy is not influenced by near total thyroidectomy: a case-control study. Clin Endocrinol (Oxf). 1999;51(4):503–8. https://doi.org/10.1046/j.1365-2265.1999.00843.x.

16. Samuels MH, Kolobova I, Niederhausen M, Janowsky JS, Schuff KG. Effects of altering levothyroxine (L-T4) doses on quality of life, mood, and cognition in L-T4 treated subjects. J Clin Endocrinol Metab. 2018;103(5):1997–2008. https://doi.org/10.1210/jc.2017-02668.

17. Godlee F. Evidence based medicine: flawed system but still the best we've got. BMJ. 2014;348:g440.

18. Else H, Van Noorden R. The fight against fake-paper factories that churn out sham science. Nature. 2021;591(7851):516–9. https://doi.org/10.1038/d41586-021-00733-5.
19. Else H. Multimillion-dollar trade in paper authorships alarms publishers. Nature. 2023;613(7945):617–8. https://doi.org/10.1038/d41586-023-00062-9.
20. Van Nuland SE, Rogers KA. Academic nightmares: predatory publishing. Anat Sci Educ. 2017;10(4):392–4. https://doi.org/10.1002/ase.1671.
21. Bagues M, Sylos-Labini M, Zinovyeva N. A walk on the wild side: 'predatory' journals and information asymmetries in scientific evaluations. Res Policy. 2017;48:462–77.
22. SCIgen. https://en.wikipedia.org/wiki/SCIgen.
23. Strielkowski W. Predatory journals: Beall's list is missed. Nature. 2017;544(7651):416. https://doi.org/10.1038/544416b.
24. Bloudoff-Indelicato M. Backlash after frontiers journals added to list of questionable publishers. Nature. 2015;526:613.
25. CabellsBlacklist. https://www2.cabells.com/about-blacklist.
26. DeVito NJ, Goldacre B. Catalogue of bias: publication bias. BMJ Evid Based Med. 2019;24(2):53–4. https://doi.org/10.1136/bmjebm-2018-111107.
27. Jefferson T. Sponsorship bias in clinical trials: growing menace or dawning realisation? J R Soc Med. 2020;113(4):148–57. https://doi.org/10.1177/0141076820914242.
28. Subbiah V, Kreitman RJ, Wainberg ZA, et al. Dabrafenib and Trametinib treatment in patients with locally advanced or metastatic BRAF V600-mutant anaplastic thyroid cancer. J Clin Oncol. 2018;36(1):7–13. https://doi.org/10.1200/JCO.2017.73.6785.
29. Smith TJ, Kahaly GJ, Ezra DG, et al. Teprotumumab for thyroid-associated ophthalmopathy. N Engl J Med. 2017;376(18):1748–61. https://doi.org/10.1056/NEJMoa1614949.
30. Mauri G, Hegedus L, Cazzato RL, Papini E. Minimally invasive treatment procedures have come of age for thyroid malignancy: the 2021 clinical practice guideline for the use of minimally invasive treatments in malignant thyroid lesions. Cardiovasc Intervent Radiol. 2021;44(9):1481–4. https://doi.org/10.1007/s00270-021-02870-w.
31. Grani G, Sponziello M, Pecce V, Ramundo V, Durante C. Contemporary thyroid nodule evaluation and management. J Clin Endocrinol Metab. 2020;105(9):2869–83. https://doi.org/10.1210/clinem/dgaa322.
32. CancerResearch_ChildhoodCancerSurvival. https://www.cancerresearchuk.org/health-professional/cancer-statistics/childrens-cancers/survival.
33. EvidenceBasedMedicineMatters. https://en.testingtreatments.org/wp-content/uploads/2016/11/Evidence-Based-Medicine-Matters.pdf.

Part II

The Manual

4

Mining the Truth

'While being well-informed about health is helpful for patients and carers, the use of the Internet and health apps by patients is associated with risks'.

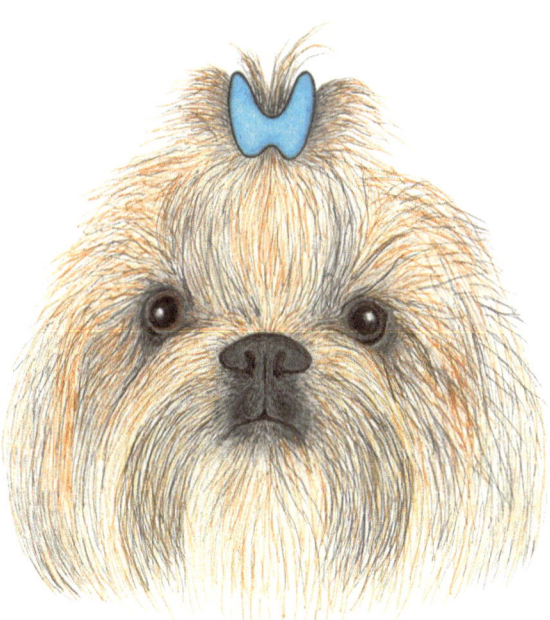

Some dog breeds are susceptible to autoimmune thyroiditis. Tests for thyroid autoantibodies have been developed, but a recent appraisal of the evidence showed that the data were poor, unreliable and unhelpful in making a diagnosis of autoimmune thyroid disease in dogs [1]

© The Author(s), under exclusive license to Springer Nature Switzerland AG 2024
P. Perros, *Seeking Thyroid Truths*, Copernicus Books,
https://doi.org/10.1007/978-3-031-58287-5_4

Nearly There

You have had to go over a lot of preliminaries so far. Your search can now commence, but you need to mind your step. This chapter will guide you in finding the sources of information that can answer your questions.

Academic Search Engines

Most health sciences academics choose to use one or more of four main portals: PubMed [2], Web of Science [3], Scopus [4] and Google Scholar [5]. The first three have relatively strict quality criteria for inclusion (e.g. a requirement for peer review of the publications that are cited). Google Scholar's main criterion is journal articles with a minimum of the abstract (summary) being freely available but includes publications that are not peer reviewed. PubMed focuses on health sciences, while the others are broader in scope.

PubMed and Google Scholar are free and serve most academics' needs well. These publications databases are designed for experts, that is, people who already have knowledge about their subject of interest and are able to choose appropriate keywords and navigate effectively. They do not work well for the unaided lay person who is likely to quickly become lost, especially if the search is general.

Searches by Patients and Lay People

The Upsides

We are increasingly turning to the Internet for health information. There is some evidence that this can be a good thing, as knowledge gained through the Internet may improve communications between the patient and doctor and facilitate decision-making [6, 7].

The Downsides

While being well-informed about health is helpful for patients and carers, the use of the Internet and health apps by patients is associated with risks. A systematic review found that the use of social media had some benefits for some people but was also associated with 'diminished subjective well-being, addiction to social media, loss of privacy and being targeted for promotion' [7]. A prospective randomised controlled study in Germany recruited students who volunteered to be subjected to unpleasant symptoms. They were then instructed to 'google' the causes of their symptoms, use a health app that provided answers about the causes of symptoms or do nothing (the latter was the 'control group' for comparison). The use of the Internet and the health app was associated with more negative behavioural effects, including more anxiety, than the control group [8]. This confirmed previous observational studies, indicating an association between health-related internet use, anxiety and depression [9–11].

Several studies have shown that anxiety and depression are associated with both hypothyroidism and hyperthyroidism, although whether this relationship is causal or not is unknown [12–15]. Specifically looking for interpretations of symptoms of hypothyroidism on Google like 'tiredness' or 'brain fog' soon brings up cancer, multiple sclerosis and dementia as possible diagnoses. This cannot be a good thing for thyroid patients who seem to be already more frequently burdened by anxiety and depression than the rest of the population. The above considerations raise the important question of whether people with thyroid disease should be encouraged to seek health information on the Internet by themselves.

Misinformation is a major concern about health-related searches on the web. This has recently led the US Surgeon General to assign 'major priority to confronting health misinformation' [16]. Here are some example of misinformation on thyroid-related topics. A survey of websites on thyroid surgery showed that 45% contained at least one inaccuracy [17]. Bogus cures for hypothyroidism are widely advertised on the Internet [18] and embellished with pseudoscience [19]. A patient website [20] quotes a study by Warren et al. (2004) [21] in support of claims that 'the lower end of the normal or reference range for TSH lies between 0.2 and 0.4 mU/L, as indicated by a number of clinical studies' and 'the TSH test is insufficient to diagnose all forms of hypothyroidism, including the borderline forms'. I can assert categorically that the study by Warren et al. is irrelevant to both claims. How can I be so sure? Not only have I read this paper, but I was one of the authors. Although in this example, misinformation was probably harmless, sometimes Internet misinformation on thyroid disease can have catastrophic effects [22].

The conclusion must be that trawling the Internet looking for evidence on thyroid-related topics, especially for causes of symptoms may be helpful to some, but it can also be overwhelming, cause negative emotional responses and lead you down rabbit holes. So, what can you do to avoid this? The answer is don't do this without some proper guidance.

Where to Start?

The best option is to perform the search under the supervision of a trustworthy expert. You can start with the doctor or nurse who is involved with managing the thyroid problem. They should be able to provide verbal and often printed information and direct you to other reliable sources. I am well aware that many thyroid patients feel that this avenue is not productive. In a UK-based survey of hypothyroid patients, only 14.5% of respondents reported being fully informed by their family doctor [23]. However, asking does not hurt, and the request can be more effective in my experience, if it is made formally in writing.

Several academic and professional organisations of experts and some patient organisations have dedicated a lot of time and effort to providing good quality material [24–28]. Some (e.g. the British Thyroid Foundation) offer an option for the user to send in their specific query, which is then answered by vetted medical advisors. There are many more, and a number of non-profit authoritative organisations have produced criteria, which identify websites with good quality information. They include the Health on the Net Foundation Code of Conduct (HONcode) [29], and the *Journal of the American Medical Association (JAMA)* benchmarks [30].

In summary, a website with good quality information should have specific characteristics [29, 30]:

- It should provide information about user privacy and confidentiality and be compliant with data protection legislation.
- It should provide information about website ownership and affiliations, funding and sponsorship.
- It should provide dates of posting of content and updates.
- The qualifications and affiliations of the authors should be given.
- Sources of information should be cited.
- The intention should be that the information is to support, not replace the medical consultation.
- Any claims in the content should be justified and supported by objective and rational thinking.
- Requests for payment and attempts to sell products through the website should make you cautious.

The above criteria will not guarantee that those websites that fulfil them are necessarily reliable, and some reliable ones may not fulfil all the conditions, but they will limit the probability of being entangled in scams and will increase the chance of accessing good quality information.

Avoiding Rabbit Holes

Searching without a clear idea of what you looking for is a recipe for getting lost and wasting time or worse ending up being misinformed. It is imperative that before the search begins, you should try to formulate as precisely as possible the question that is to be answered. If you are wondering whether you have an underactive thyroid, then the relevant question may be 'how is hypothyroidism diagnosed?'

Seeking Specific Information About the Thyroid: The Shortcut Route

One way of answering the question 'how is hypothyroidism diagnosed?' is to take a shortcut to authoritative professional organisations that produce guidelines, consensus statements or position statements on thyroid topics. Below is a list of such professional organisations and the topics covered, with citations that will lead you to the relevant source (Table 4.1). A 'citation' or 'reference' is the description of a published piece of academic work and usually includes

Table 4.1 Authoritative professional organisations that produce guidelines, consensus statements or position statements on thyroid topics

- British Thyroid Association (hypothyroidism, thyrotoxicosis, thyroid cancer) [31, 32]
- National Institute for Health and Care Excellence (hypothyroidism, thyrotoxicosis, thyroid cancer) [33, 34]
- Society for Endocrinology (hypothyroidism) [35]
- British Association of Endocrine and Thyroid Surgeons (thyroid surgery) [36]
- British Society of Paediatric Endocrinology and Diabetes (thyroid nodules and cancer in children) [37]
- Royal College of Physicians (thyroid eye disease) [38]
- European Thyroid Association (23 guidelines/consensus statements on various thyroid topics) [39]
- American Thyroid Association (20 guidelines/consensus statements on various thyroid topics) [40]
- American Association of Clinical Endocrinologists (hypothyroidism, hyperthyroidism, thyroid nodules) [41]
- European Society For Medical Oncology (thyroid cancer) [42]
- National Comprehensive Cancer Network (thyroid cancer) [43]
- European Association of Nuclear Medicine (thyroid cancer) [44]
- Cochrane library (59 systematic reviews on various thyroid topics) [45]
- BMJ evidence (several thyroid topics; requires subscription) [46]
- UpToDate (several thyroid topics; requires subscription) [47]
- Dynamed (several thyroid topics; requires subscription) [48]

the names of the authors, the title of the work, the name of the journal (or book, or website), year, issue number and page number.

Such publications as those derived from organisations shown above are likely to have answers to your questions and will cite the primary sources of information that their conclusions are based on. For example, in relation to the question 'how is hypothyroidism diagnosed', the National Institute for Health and Care Excellence guideline 'Thyroid disease: assessment and management' [33] includes a document labelled '1.2 Investigating suspected thyroid dysfunction or thyroid enlargement'. The information contained there states that the relevant blood tests are TSH, free T4 and free T3. It also has a link to a detailed explanation on where the evidence comes from: 'evidence review C: thyroid function tests' [33], which lists seven relevant sources:

- Brochmann H, Bjoro T, Gaarder PI, Hanson F, Frey HM. Prevalence of thyroid dysfunction in elderly subjects. A randomized study in a Norwegian rural community (Naeroy). Acta Endocrinol. 1988;117(1):7–12.
- Feldkamp CS, Carey JL. An algorithmic approach to thyroid function testing in a managed care setting. 3-year experience. Am J Clin Pathol. 1996;105(1):11–6.
- Henze M, Brown SJ, Hadlow NC, Walsh JP. Rationalizing thyroid function testing: which TSH cutoffs are optimal for testing free T4? J Clin Endocrinol Metab. 2017;102(11):4235–4241.
- Koulouri O, Gurnell M. How to interpret thyroid function tests. Clin Med. 2013;13(3):282–6.
- National Institute for Health and Care Excellence. Developing NICE guidelines: the manual [updated October 2018]. London: National Institute for Health and Care Excellence; 2014. http://www.nice.org.uk/article/PMG20/chapter/1%20Introduction%20and%20overview.
- Notas G, Kampa M, Malliaraki N, Petrodaskalaki M, Papavasileiou S, Castanas E. Implementation of thyroid function tests algorithms by clinical laboratories: a four-year experience of good clinical and diagnostic practice in a tertiary hospital in Greece. Eur J Intern Med. 2018;54:81–86.
- Snabboon T, Sridama V, Sunthornyothin S, Suwanwalaikorn S, Vongthavaravat V. A more appropriate algorithm of thyroid function test in diagnosis of hyperthyroidism for Thai patients. J Med Assoc Thailand. 2004;87(Suppl 2):S19–S21.

Beware though that the National Institute for Health and Care Excellence document [33], as stated on the front page when you access it, was published in 2019; therefore, publications on the topic since 2019 are not included. To get up-to-date publications, you will need to do more searches.

Using Academic Search Engines for Primary Publications

If the sources from authoritative professional organisations listed earlier have not produced an answer, you can use one of the free academic search engines mentioned at the start of this chapter.

PubMed [2] is a popular search engine, and here, I will provide an example of how I would use PubMed to find answers to 'how is hypothyroidism diagnosed'. Before using PubMed, I would strongly recommend that you spend a bit of time reading the PubMed User guide [49], which will also direct you to some very useful tutorials. You can search PubMed for a topic using phrases or keywords. My preference is to use keywords and I enter 'hypothyroidism' and 'diagnosis' (without the quotation marks) in the search box. This produces nearly 30,000 hits. Now I would use filters to make the search more focused. Using filters to restrict to 'humans', 'English language' and last '10 years' since publication yields about 3500 publications. These are ranked in order of highest relevance to the search terms.

So, now I can pick the top 50 or so and browse through. I can immediately pick nine references from the top 50 that look highly promising (citations marked as * are freely available in full text).

- Wilson SA, et al. Hypothyroidism: diagnosis and treatment. Am Fam Physician. 2021;103(10):605–613.
- Duntas LH, Yen PM. Diagnosis and treatment of hypothyroidism in the elderly. Endocrine. 2019;66(1):63–69.
- *Chiovato L, et al. Hypothyroidism in context: where we've been and where we're going. Adv Ther. 2019;36(Suppl 2):47–58.
- *Calissendorff J, Falhammar H. To treat or not to treat subclinical hypothyroidism, what is the evidence? Medicina (Kaunas). 2020;56(1):40.
- Dunn D, Turner C. Hypothyroidism in women. Nurs Womens Health. 2016;20(1):93–8.
- Peeters RP. Subclinical hypothyroidism. N Engl J Med. 2017;376(26):2556–2565.
- Gottwald-Hostalek U, Schulte B. Low awareness and under-diagnosis of hypothyroidism. Curr Med Res Opin. 2022;38(1):59–64.
- Garmendia Madariaga A, et al. The incidence and prevalence of thyroid dysfunction in Europe: a meta-analysis. J Clin Endocrinol Metab. 2014;99(3):923–31.
- Siskind SM, et al. Investigating hypothyroidism. BMJ. 2021;373:n993.

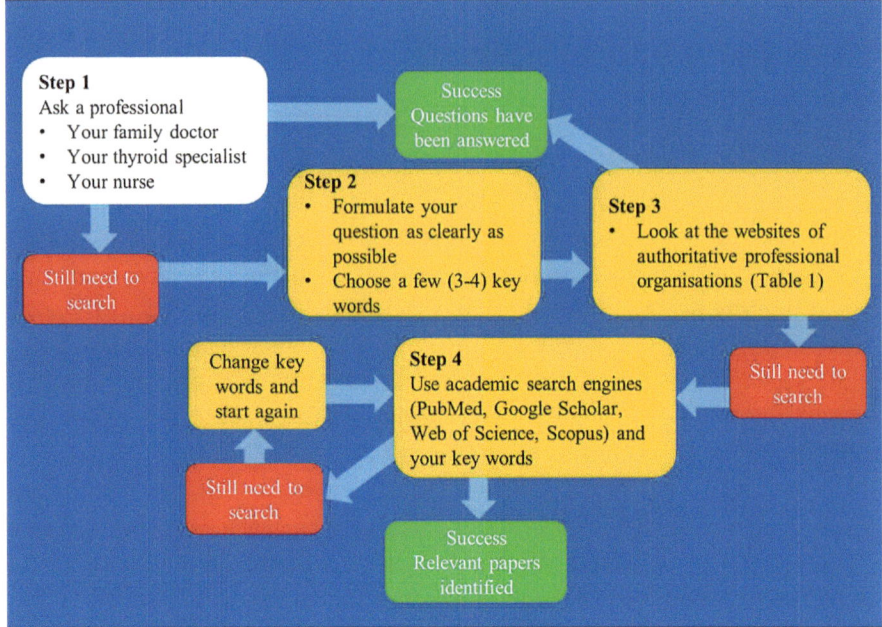

Fig. 4.1 Summary of the initial search strategy

You may have noticed that all of the above are reviews rather than primary sources of evidence; however, they will cite the primary sources. A similar search in Google Scholar will yield some additional references (as the search methods and filters are not identical to PubMed), so conducting the same searches in both search engines may be fruitful. A summary of how to go about with your initial search is shown in Fig. 4.1.

Other Types of Searches

If you already have the full citation for a reference, then any search engine will likely lead you to the abstract and if you are lucky to the full text. You can also search by the title of a publication or by the name of a particular author [50].

Accessing Full-Text Publications

Assuming that you now have some citations, it is possible to (at the very least) access the abstract (summary) of the publication. PubMed will bring the abstract up if you double click on the citation. The abstract will be quite informative and helps to confirm that it is (or is not) relevant to your question that is being explored.

Most citations on PubMed and Google Scholar have links to the full text of the paper, and in a sizeable proportion, it is possible to access or download the whole article free of charge. Others unfortunately have restricted access or 'paywalls'. There are several avenues worth exploring if you wish to access the full text without paying or at a low cost. Public libraries may be able to request a reprint with a minimal charge. If you belong to academic institutions or health organisations, you may automatically have access. Sometimes you can access papers through ResearchGate [51]. Or you can contact the corresponding author (a Google search by the name and the institution as it appears in the abstract often brings up an email address) and ask for the pdf. Internet Archive Scholar [52] is also worth a try. Sci-Hub is described as '*a shadow library website that provides free access to millions of research papers and books, without regard to copyright, by bypassing publishers' paywalls in various ways*' [53]. I have never used it because of the lack of clarity over its legal status and am unable to comment on its utility. The same applies to unpaywall.org, paperpanda.app, 12ft.io and openaccessbutton.org. A summary of how to access full-text publications in shown in Fig. 4.2.

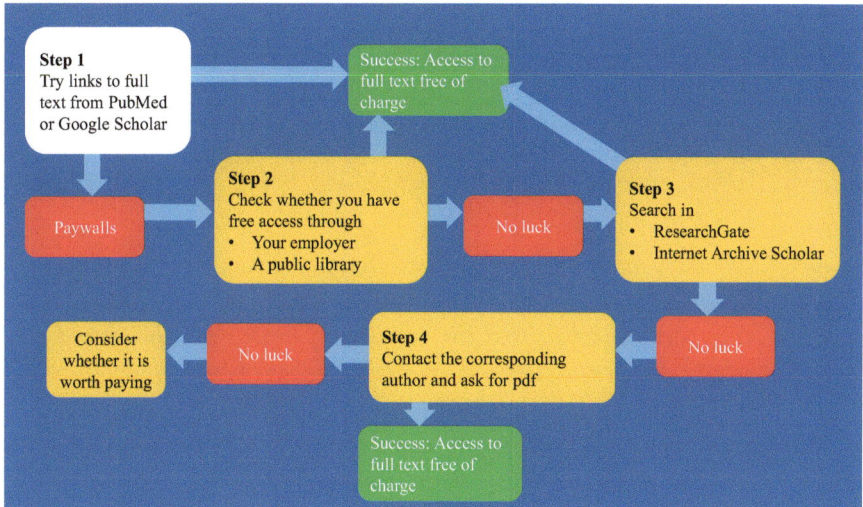

Fig. 4.2 Summary of how to access full-text publications

Red Flags in Conducting Searches

If the sources quoted above are used, you are unlikely to encounter 'dodgy' websites; however, if you use general search engines such as Google, you almost certainly will. You should be very cautious about websites that include aggressive advertising or trying to sell something or demand payment for services.

Look out for emotional language, which usually signifies partiality and bias. You should not trust opinions that are not based on evidence or when validity is claimed simply because many others concur. And beware of conspiracy theorists.

What About ChatGPT?

If you ask ChatGPT 'how is hypothyroidism diagnosed?' you will get the following answer:

Hypothyroidism is typically diagnosed through a combination of medical history, physical examination, and blood tests to measure thyroid hormone levels. During a physical exam, the doctor will check for signs and symptoms of hypothyroidism, such as dry skin, hair loss, slowed reflexes, and swelling in the neck (enlarged thyroid gland). Blood tests are used to measure the levels of thyroid-stimulating hormone (TSH) and thyroxine (T4) in the blood. TSH is produced by the pituitary gland and stimulates the thyroid gland to produce T4, which is then converted to the active thyroid hormone, tri-iodothyronine (T3). In hypothyroidism, the TSH level is typically elevated because the pituitary gland is trying to stimulate the thyroid gland to produce more thyroid hormones. Meanwhile, the T4 level is usually low because the thyroid gland is not producing enough hormones. Other tests, such as thyroid antibody tests, may be done to determine if the hypothyroidism is caused by an autoimmune disorder, such as Hashimoto's thyroiditis. It's important to note that the diagnosis of hypothyroidism should always be made by a healthcare professional, and self-diagnosis based on symptoms alone is not recommended.

You can ask ChatGPT to reveal its sources by asking 'please provide sources for the previous answer'. This is what comes up:

1. American Thyroid Association. Hypothyroidism. 2017. https://www.thyroid.org/hypothyroidism/.
2. Mayo Clinic. Hypothyroidism (underactive thyroid). 2021. https://www.mayoclinic.org/diseases-conditions/hypothyroidism/diagnosis-treatment/drc-20350289.
3. National Institute of Diabetes and Digestive and Kidney Diseases. Hypothyroidism (underactive thyroid). 2021. https://www.niddk.nih.gov/health-information/endocrine-diseases/hypothyroidism.

I am cautiously impressed by ChatGPT in that at least the sources cited comply with criteria for good-quality websites. The American bias is of course obvious, and the sources do not include publications in the medical literature. Many concerns have been voiced about the performance of ChatGPT, but for sure, AI is going to get better.

A taste of what is around the corner with regard to AI is provided by a recent study published in the in JAMA Internal Medicine (impact factor 44.4). It compared responses of qualified physicians to medical questions posted on Reddit, with responses generated by ChatGPT [54]. The ChatGPT responses were not only of better quality but also more empathetic than those of the physicians.

So hopefully you have succeeded in finding some relevant answers to your question and with some luck one or more free full-text publications. No cause for celebrations yet, as you will find out in the next chapter.

References

1. Treeful AE, Coffey EL, Friedenberg SG. A scoping review of autoantibodies as biomarkers for canine autoimmune disease. J Vet Intern Med. 2022;36(2):363–78. https://doi.org/10.1111/jvim.16392.
2. PubMed. https://pubmed.ncbi.nlm.nih.gov/.
3. Web of Science. https://clarivate.com/webofsciencegroup/solutions/web-of-science/.
4. Scopus. https://www.scopus.com/.

5. GoogleScholar. https://scholar.google.co.uk/.
6. Tan SS, Goonawardene N. Internet health information seeking and the patient-physician relationship: a systematic review. J Med Internet Res. 2017;19(1):e9. https://doi.org/10.2196/jmir.5729.
7. Smailhodzic E, Hooijsma W, Boonstra A, Langley DJ. Social media use in healthcare: a systematic review of effects on patients and on their relationship with healthcare professionals. BMC Health Serv Res. 2016;16(1):442. https://doi.org/10.1186/s12913-016-1691-0.
8. Jungmann SM, Brand S, et al. Do Dr. Google and health apps have (comparable) side effects? An experimental study. Clin Psychol Sci. 2020;8(2):306–17.
9. Bessiere K, Pressman S, Kiesler S, Kraut R. Effects of internet use on health and depression: a longitudinal study. J Med Internet Res. 2010;12(1):e6. https://doi.org/10.2196/jmir.1149.
10. Singh K, Brown RJ. From headache to tumour: an examination of health anxiety, health-related internet use and 'query escalation'. J Health Psychol. 2016;21(9):2008–20. https://doi.org/10.1177/1359105315569620.
11. Wangler J, Jansky M. Internetassoziierte Gesundheitsangste in der hausarztlichen Versorgung—Ergebnisse einer Befragung unter Allgemeinmedizinern und hausarztlich tatigen Internisten in Hessen [Internet-associated health anxieties in primary care—results of a survey among general practitioners and primary care internists in Hesse]. Dtsch Med Wochenschr. 2019;144(16):e102–e108. https://doi.org/10.1055/a-0842-8285.
12. Siegmann EM, Muller HHO, Luecke C, Philipsen A, Kornhuber J, Gromer TW. Association of depression and anxiety disorders with autoimmune thyroiditis: a systematic review and meta-analysis. JAMA Psychiatry. 2018;75(6):577–84. https://doi.org/10.1001/jamapsychiatry.2018.0190.
13. Brandt F, Thvilum M, Almind D, et al. Hyperthyroidism and psychiatric morbidity: evidence from a Danish nationwide register study. Eur J Endocrinol. 2014;170(2):341–8. https://doi.org/10.1530/EJE-13-0708.
14. Thvilum M, Brandt F, Almind D, Christensen K, Brix TH, Hegedus L. Increased psychiatric morbidity before and after the diagnosis of hypothyroidism: a nationwide register study. Thyroid. 2014;24(5):802–8. https://doi.org/10.1089/thy.2013.0555.
15. Bove KB, Watt T, Vogel A, et al. Anxiety and depression are more prevalent in patients with Graves' disease than in patients with nodular goitre. Eur Thyroid J. 2014;3(3):173–8. https://doi.org/10.1159/000365211.
16. USSurgeonGeneral. Confronting health misinformation: the US Surgeon General's advisory on building a healthy information environment. 2021. Publications and reports of the Surgeon General.
17. Harper C, Bonner A, Alexander A, et al. Down the rabbit hole: evaluation of internet information quality in parathyroid and thyroid surgery. J Surg Res. 2023;282:65–70. https://doi.org/10.1016/j.jss.2022.09.004.

18. BogusCures. https://www.buzzfeednews.com/article/carolinehaskins1/sea-moss-does-not-cure-thyroid-disease-but-people-sell-it.
19. Pseudoscience. https://sciencebasedmedicine.org/hypothyroidism-the-facts-the-controversies-and-the-pseudoscience/.
20. TPAUK_1. https://www.tpauk.com/main/article/studiesresearch-doubts-on-the-usefulness-of-serumtsh-and-free-t4-testing-which-are-being-ignored/.
21. Warren RE, Perros P, Nyirenda MJ, Frier BM. Serum thyrotropin is a better predictor of future thyroid dysfunction than thyroid autoantibody status in biochemically euthyroid patients with diabetes: implications for screening. Thyroid. 2004;14(10):853–7. https://doi.org/10.1089/thy.2004.14.853.
22. Neuberg GW, Stephenson KE, Sears DA, McConnell RJ. Internet-enabled thyroid hormone abuse. Ann Intern Med. 2009;150(1):60–1. https://doi.org/10.7326/0003-4819-150-1-200901060-00021.
23. Mitchell AL, Hegedus L, Zarkovic M, Hickey JL, Perros P. Patient satisfaction and quality of life in hypothyroidism: an online survey by the British Thyroid Foundation. Clin Endocrinol (Oxf). 2021;94(3):513–20. https://doi.org/10.1111/cen.14340.
24. BritishThyroidAssociationPatientResources. https://www.british-thyroid-association.org/services-3#patientresources.
25. BritishThyroidFoundation. https://www.btf-thyroid.org/.
26. AmericanThyroidAssociationPatientInformation. https://www.thyroid.org/thyroid-information/.
27. ButterflyThyroidCancerTrust.
28. YouAndYourHormones. https://www.yourhormones.info/.
29. HeathOnTheNet. https://www.hon.ch/en/about.html
30. Winker MA, Flanagin A, Chi-Lum B, et al. Guidelines for medical and health information sites on the internet: principles governing AMA web sites. American Medical Association. JAMA. 2000;283(12):1600–6. https://doi.org/10.1001/jama.283.12.1600.
31. Ahluwalia R, Baldeweg SE, Boelaert K, et al. Use of liothyronine (T3) in hypothyroidism: joint British Thyroid Association/Society for Endocrinology consensus statement. Clin Endocrinol (Oxf). 2023;99(2):206–16. https://doi.org/10.1111/cen.14935.
32. BTAGuidelines. https://www.british-thyroid-association.org/current-bta-guidelines-and-statements.
33. NICEThyroidFunctionTests. https://www.nice.org.uk/guidance/ng145/evidence/c-thyroid-function-tests-pdf-6967421679.
34. NICEThyroidCancer. https://www.nice.org.uk/guidance/ng230.
35. SfEGuidelines. https://www.endocrinology.org/clinical-practice/clinical-guidance/society-position-statements/.
36. BAETSGuidelines. BAETSGuidelines. https://www.baets.org.uk/guidelines/.
37. BSPEDGuidelines. BSPEDGuidelines. https://www.bsped.org.uk/media/1373/rareendocrinetumour_final.pdf.

38. Perros P, Dayan CM, Dickinson AJ, et al. Management of patients with Graves' orbitopathy: initial assessment, management outside specialised centres and referral pathways. Clin Med (Lond). 2015;15(2):173–8. https://doi.org/10.7861/clinmedicine.15-2-173.
39. ETAGuidelines. https://www.eurothyroid.com/guidelines/eta_guidelines.html.
40. ATAGuidelines. https://www.thyroid.org/professionals/ata-professional-guidelines/.
41. AACEGuidelines. https://pro.aace.com/resources?keys=&disease_state_resource_cat_1%5Bthyroid%5D=thyroid&field_disease_state_content_t_value%5BGuidelines%5D=Guidelines.
42. ESMOGuidelines. https://www.esmo.org/guidelines/guidelines-by-topic/endocrine-and-neuroendocrine-cancers/thyroid-cancer.
43. NCCNGuidelines. https://www.nccn.org/guidelines/guidelines-detail?category=1&id=1470.
44. EANMGuidelines. https://www.eanm.org/publications/guidelines/endocrine-system/.
45. CochraneLibrary. https://www.cochranelibrary.com/.
46. BMJEvidence. https://bestpractice.bmj.com/evidence.
47. UptoDate. https://www.uptodate.com/login.
48. Dytnamed. https://www.dynamed.com/.
49. PubMedUserGuide. https://pubmed.ncbi.nlm.nih.gov/help/.
50. PubMedAuthor. https://pubmed.ncbi.nlm.nih.gov/help/#author-search.
51. ResearchGate. https://www.researchgate.net/.
52. InternetArchiveScholar. InternetArchiveScholar. https://scholar.archive.org/.
53. Sci-Hub. https://en.wikipedia.org/wiki/Sci-Hub.
54. Ayers JW, Poliak A, Dredze M, et al. Comparing physician and artificial intelligence Chatbot responses to patient questions posted to a public social media forum. JAMA Intern Med. 2023;183(6):589–96. https://doi.org/10.1001/jamainternmed.2023.1838.

5

Appraising the Evidence

'Papers that have not been peer reviewed are suspect and probably not worth reading'.

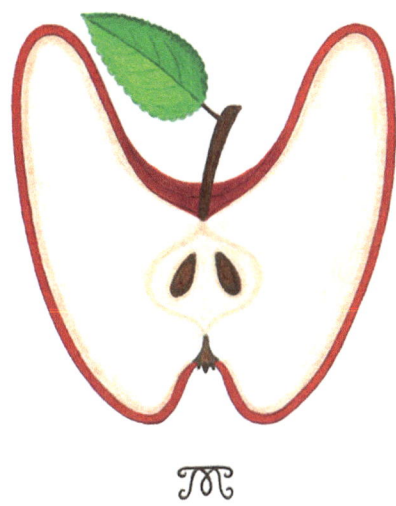

Shortcut or Long-Way Round

You may have reached this point the long way round, having searched PubMed or Google Scholar and succeeded in identifying one or more original publications that are relevant to the questions that you have in mind. Now you need to decide how good the evidence is. Or you may have taken a shortcut and found your answer in a narrative review, systematic review, meta-analysis, guideline or consensus statement, which will have appraised the evidence for you. If you are satisfied with the interpretation given by such secondary publications, you have reached your destination.

One important caveat is that knowledge evolves rapidly, and if your source is more than 4–5 years old, there may be newer evidence that could overturn the conclusions of the old, which is why guidelines are often revised. For example, UK guidelines on the treatment of thyroid cancer were first published in 2002 [1] and were revised in 2007 [2], 2014 [3] and 2022 [4], in order to keep abreast of the evolving evidence. Also, narrative reviews, systematic reviews, meta-analyses, guidelines or consensus statements do not always get it right (though that is rare). There will always therefore be a need to decide for yourself if the evidence you have unearthed is of good quality.

Good Eggs, Bad Eggs

This chapter focuses on appraising original (primary) pieces of research from a 'checklist' perspective in the same way that pilots do before take-off and landing. Pilot checklists do not guarantee that the flight will be smooth or trouble-free, but serious problems are usually picked up, and this practice has improved aviation safety. In a similar way, there are criteria in relation to medical publications that, if met, increase the probability of good quality and conversely their absence should raise doubts.

The aim of this chapter is to introduce you to this checklist, which will help sort the bad eggs from the rest. This is a challenge as no set of simple rules can do this reliably. However, there are benchmarks that can be used and that is what this chapter is about.

A Word of Warning

Some of the criteria outlined below may not apply to old publications (those published more than 20 years ago), as research was not as regulated as it is today. One such example is a paper by Braverman and Ingbar published in

1970, which confirmed that levothyroxine was converted by peripheral tissues in humans to the active thyroid hormone tri-iodothyronine (T3) [5]. Several items on the checklist are not fulfilled (e.g. no mention of ethical approval, no study oversight or study registration). Yet, this was one of the most important studies in the field and set the foundations upon which other discoveries were made.

Starting with the Abstract

At this point, you should be able to access the abstract of papers free of charge. As long as you have the citation, a search on PubMed or Google Scholar or just Google should bring up the abstract, which usually is pretty short (200–300 words). This minimal information is usually enough to work out whether it is worth reading the entire article or not.

Have You Hit the Target?

Once you have read the abstract, it should be obvious whether the contents are relevant to the question that you have in mind. If not, it is probably best to leave it at that and move on.

Has the Study Been Superseded?

Studies that are several years old may no longer be valid because newer more robust research has superseded them or they were so perfect that nobody can do better, which is as unusual as unicorns. So, you should be cautious about old citations.

A clue will be the number of times the study has been cited since its publication and especially whether it continues to be cited. Such information can be found in Google Scholar (underneath each hit, there will be a note 'cited by' followed by a number). Studies that are of mediocre quality are forgotten, while the real unicorns are cited time and time again. Watson and Crick's paper on the structure of DNA in 1953 [6] has been cited 17,570 times, including 330 times in the first 6 months of 2023, according to Google Scholar. A case report about thyroid eye disease published in the same year as the Watson and Crick paper has attracted in total 16 citations and none in the first 6 months of 2023 [7]. This of course is not a perfect way to judge whether a paper is time-expired, as there are anomalies. For example, a paper published in 1998, which was subsequently retracted, has been cited 4292 times, not for its scientific merit, but because of its notoriety and as an example of bad science [8]. Note that papers published within the past 12 months may not be cited much despite being of high quality, as it takes time for a newly published paper to be read and for subsequent papers to cite it.

As mentioned in the previous chapter, not all of the citations in Google Scholar are peer-reviewed. The most reliable means of finding out how many times a paper has been cited by other peer-reviewed journals is Scopus [9], but unfortunately, you need to be a subscriber. So, for the majority of people wishing to find out how often a paper has been cited, Google Scholar is the main option, which is a reasonable approximation to citations in other peer-reviewed papers.

Checklists

I have divided the checklists into Simple and Advanced. The Simple Checklist is for everyone who has access to the Internet and is based on information that appears in the paper abstract. It is easier to use, but less reliable than the Advanced Appraisal Checklist and should be regarded as a screening test for quality. For those who are unable to proceed to the Advanced Appraisal Checklist, I have included some items in the Simple Checklist under the heading 'Collateral evidence that can be used to shape an opinion about the quality of the paper'. The Advanced Appraisal Checklist is more complicated and requires getting your hands on the full-text paper.

Red Flag

Beware of publications in journals that are not peer reviewed. You can check by looking for the paper in PubMed [10], Web of Science [11] or Scopus [9]. If it appears in these databases, it is almost certain that it has been peer reviewed. You can also search the journal website and confirm that there is a mandatory peer-review process in place before publication.

Papers that have not been peer reviewed are suspect and probably not worth reading. Here is an example. A publication by L Pollack is cited by Google Scholar [12], but the journal is not peer reviewed and it shows. The author, using an individual case, tries to argue that thyroid overactivity can be treated successfully with homeopathy. The fact that the patient was also treated by her physician with anti-thyroid drugs is conveniently overlooked.

Green Flag

Two or more independent studies with similar conclusions, in the absence of studies with contradictory findings, make it very likely that the results should be taken seriously, assuming that the Checklists do not identify serious flaws.

> **Simple Appraisal Checklist for Quality of Publications**
> - The paper is not a case report.
> - The publication has been peer reviewed.
> - There is a clearly stated study aim.
> - The study design is described.
> - The results are presented clearly and supported by statistical analyses.
> - The conclusions are grounded on the results.
> - Collateral evidence.
>   - *Impact factor*
>   - *Author affiliations and scholarly metrics*
>   - *Citations*

Notes for Simple Appraisal Checklist

The Paper Is Not a Case Report

Case reports may contain information that can identify an interesting direction for further research but are extremely unlikely to provide sufficient evidence for drawing conclusions. For this reason, case reports are unreliable and should be dismissed, as the risk of bias is very high.

Has the Paper Been Peer-Reviewed?

If not, this is a red flag (see above).

Is There a Clearly Stated Aim?

The aim of a study should be stated in the abstract. It is important that this is well described and it should be crystal clear what the research question is (what is it about, what type of subject or patient it is about; what is being compared with what, if it is about treatment what the treatment is; and what are the outcomes that are measured).

Examples A **poor example** is Tang et al. [13] The paper is about 'Hashimoto's encephalopathy', but the abstract does not inform the reader at all about what the investigators were trying to address. A **good example** is a paper by Gussekloo and colleagues [14], where the abstract states that the aim was to find out whether elderly people with mild untreated hypothyroidism live as long as people with normal thyroid tests and whether they suffer greater disability, depression and memory loss.

What Is the Study Design?

The abstract should describe the study design (e.g. case report, observational, randomised etc.). If this information is lacking, it is probably not worth reading.

Examples Here is a **poor example** claiming that ozone treatment benefits women with hypothyroidism and infertility [15]. The abstract states that two groups of women were compared, but there are no clues as to whether this was retrospective, prospective, randomised or blinded. A **good example** is a paper by Walsh and colleagues who conducted a study to assess whether 'fine-tuning' the dose of levothyroxine had an impact on well-being [16]. They state in the abstract 'we conducted a double-blind, randomised clinical trial with a cross-over design'. This tells us that groups of patients were allocated entirely by chance ('randomized') to have a small change in dose of levothyroxine or not, that neither the patients nor the researchers know which group was allocated to what treatment ('double-blind'), and after spending some time having one dose of levothyroxine, they were switched to receive a slightly different dose ('cross-over').

How Are the Results Presented?

The results should be presented clearly, and it should be stated whether any differences between groups are statistically significant.

Examples The 'International Journal of Ayurverda and Pharma Research' is allegedly peer reviewed and in 2019 published a study on the effects of Agnimandhya Virechana yoga in patients with hypothyroidism [17]. In this **poor example**, the results section of the abstract state: 'Effect of *Virechana karma* was seen extremely significant on symptoms like fatigue, dry and coarse skin, unexplained weight gain, muscle ache, puffiness of face and breathlessness. After the treatment, the average TSH value reduced from 153.03 to 138.41. This is observed that the TSH level was reduced up to 9.88%'. The reader is left wondering what 'extremely significant' means, in particular whether it refers to statistical significance and whether the change in TSH level from 153.03 to 138.41 is of any value to patients. A **good example** is a study that explored thyroid tests (TSH, T3, T4, reverse T3 and T2 levels) in patients with thyroid cancer on levothyroxine treatment and correlated these levels of quality of life [18]. The results section is clear and coherent. It states the values of the hormones and goes on to inform the reader that the levels of these hormones did not correlate with the quality of life according to statistical tests.

Are the Conclusions Grounded on the Results?

The conclusions must not be far-fetched or speculative and should not over-interpret and over-generalise the results.

Examples A **poor example** is a paper published in 1995, which studied 20 patients with thyroid eye disease and treated them with a drug called 'octreotide' [19]. Eight patients with thyroid eye disease served as controls (did not receive the treatment). Seven of the 20 patients treated, but none of the eight controls, showed an improvement. The authors concluded that octreotide has a beneficial effect in the thyroid eye. This study suffered from not being randomised or blinded and from the very small number of patients, but most importantly from overestimation of the validity of study, which was insufficient to support the conclusion that the drug was beneficial. Thyroid eye disease tends to get better with time even without treatment, and this was not taken into account. In the years that followed three randomised double-blind controlled trials **(good examples)** failed to show a benefit of this class of drug in thyroid eye disease [20–22].

Collateral Evidence

There are some additional indicators that may help in deciding on the quality of a paper. These are far less reliable than the Advanced Appraisal Checklist, but better than nothing if you cannot access the full text of a paper.

Impact Factor

If the impact factor of the journal is low (less than 3) or the journal has no impact factor, then the quality is likely to be poor. Impact factors are reported by journals on their website and can also be found in bioxbio (https://www.bioxbio.com/).

Examples **Poor examples:** In the 1990s, several papers were published claiming that liothyronine treatment was effective in patients with fibromyalgia in an obscure journal (Clinical Bulletin of Myofascial Therapy) with no impact factor [23–25]. **Good example**: A subsequent guideline in a journal with an impact factor of 12.3 did not recommend thyroid hormone treatment for patients with fibromyalgia [26].

Author Affiliations and Scholarly Metrics

You can look at the affiliations of the authors. It would be unusual and it should raise concerns if the authors have private addresses and are not affiliated with academic institutions.

Examples **Poor example**: A paper published in the *Journal of Nutritional & Environmental Medicine* (no impact factor) claimed that patients with normal thyroid blood tests, but with symptoms of hypothyroidism benefited from receiving levothyroxine treatment [27]. None of the authors had academic affiliations. Furthermore, the study was not controlled, so there was no comparative group. **Good example:** A randomised double-blind, placebo controlled study investigated the same question, that is whether levothyroxine in people who complain of hypothyroid-like symptoms but have normal thyroid blood tests is beneficial. All authors were affiliated with University Departments or a major teaching hospital [28]. Levothyroxine had no effect in this study.

You can check if the authors have produced other academic publications. The Hirsch index (H-index) is a metric for individual academics and is calculated on the basis of how many times that person's papers have been cited by peers. For an academic who has been working for 20 years or more, an H-index of 20 is said to be 'good', 40 is 'outstanding' and 60 is 'truly exceptional' [29]. It is not easy to find the H-index of authors unless you have access to Scopus [9] or Web of Science [11]. Some academics provide information on their H-index in their academic websites. Not all co-authors in a paper should be expected to have a respectable H-index, but having at least one author with a H-index of more than 20 is reassuring. **Poor example:** In the poor example cited above [27] the highest H-index among the authors was 21, while in the **good example** [28], one co-author had an H-index of 44.

Citations

The value of recent citations of the paper as an indirect indicator of whether a piece of research has been superseded was already discussed earlier. The number of citations of a paper is also a rough indicator of quality, although this is time-dependent, and very recent papers are unlikely to have been cited widely even if of high quality.

Examples Here is a **good example** of how collateral evidence seems to be of value: the discovery that a particular mutation on a gene called BRAF was responsible for a type of thyroid cancer was published in 2003 [30]. This was a major advance in understanding how thyroid tumours arise and has opened up new treatment avenues for thyroid cancer [31]. This paper [30] has been cited 1123 times. The impact factor of the journal is 12 and the H-index of the senior authors is 71. **Poor example:** The paper on ozone treatment in women with hypothyroidism and infertility [15] has attracted no citations since its publication in 2017, and the most senior author's H-index is 17.

Advanced Appraisal Checklist for Quality of Publications
- The way that participants were selected is described.
- The baseline characteristics of the groups of patients are comparable.
- The study has sufficient statistical power.
- Statistical tests are appropriate.
- Missing data are handled appropriately.
- In clinical trials, early stops are justified.
- The measurements are validated.
- Methods are sufficiently detailed for replication.
- Potential conflicts of interest are addressed.
- Funding information is included.
- Study oversight information is included (not applicable for studies performed more than 20–30 years ago).
- Study registration is included (not applicable for studies conducted before 2005).
- Ethical approval is addressed.
- The results of the study have been replicated by an independent group of researchers.

Notes for Advanced Appraisal Checklist

Once you have decided from the abstract that a paper is worth pursuing, you can try to lay your hands on the full text (the 'how' is described in Chapter Four under 'Accessing full text publications'). Here there are additional questions that need to be answered about quality.

How Were Participants Selected?

The methods section should provide information about how subjects were selected. This is crucial because 'selection bias' is a common and troublesome distractor.

Examples Imagine that you have to drive 100 miles for an important meeting. You can either go via route A or route B. Driving time is roughly the same, but you want to know what the chances of a major delay are for either of the two routes. You find a traffic report on Google, which states that the driving times for 1000 vehicles were measured for each of the routes and 50% were delayed via route A versus 10% via route B. This seems to be a compelling argument in favour of route B. But hidden somewhere in the small print of the report is a statement that the counts were made on one single day. It so happens that on that day there was a major accident on route A. Selection bias (by choosing to limit the counts on a single day) has provided a picture that may not be representative. To reduce selection bias, one would have to count delays on multiple days, and the more the better.

Here is an example of selection bias that relates to thyroid research. In Chap. 1, a study was mentioned that set out to explore the cause of persistent symptoms among levothyroxine-treated patients [32]. The investigators did well to derive their study population from a large number of hypothyroid patients and comparative controls from the community. Picking hypothyroid patients from a specialist thyroid clinic would almost certainly have been biased in favour of patients with persistent complaints, as this is one of the reasons why patients are referred from the community to specialists. Selecting patients from family doctor records for being prescribed levothyroxine assumed that such patients had a diagnosis of hypothyroidism, which seems fair. The investigators could have been even more meticulous and looked for documented evidence of abnormal thyroid blood tests before starting treatment that confirmed the diagnosis of hypothyroidism, but that was not done. It would have been practically more difficult, laborious and time consuming, so a shortcut was taken. The authors concluded that the study provided evidence to indicate that hypothyroid patients on levothyroxine replacement even with a normal TSH endure significant impairment in psychological well-being compared to controls of similar age and sex. This paper according to Google Scholar has been cited 630 times, in many cases as evidence that levothyroxine does not relieve the symptoms of hypothyroidism in about 15% of patients, even if the blood tests (serum TSH) are normalised. The publishers of the journal that it appeared in would be very pleased with the positive effect that this paper has had on the journal's impact factor.

Twelve years later, a study from the UK [33] showed that about 6.3% of patients being prescribed levothyroxine had normal thyroid blood tests before levothyroxine treatment was started and 58% had 'subclinical hypothyroidism', a mild disturbance of thyroid blood tests now known not to be associated with hypothyroid symptoms [34] and therefore symptom improvement with thyroid hormones is not expected any more than in people without thyroid problems. Data from the USA [35] published in 2021 showed that 30.5% of patients being prescribed levothyroxine had normal thyroid blood tests before starting treatment, and a meta-analysis revealed that in cases where the evidence for hypothyroidism before starting levothyroxine treatment was unclear, more than a third of patients were able to come off treatment without becoming hypothyroid [36].

The above data and the possible bias in selecting people with hypothyroidism raise the question of whether the estimate of patients whose symptoms are not relieved with levothyroxine in the original paper described above is accurate.

Were the Groups Comparable at Baseline?

Studies of human subjects should provide a table that lists the demographic (e.g. age, sex) and other baseline characteristics of the participants. If there are two or more groups being compared, the baseline characteristics should be similar to ensure like is compared with like and the numbers in each group should be roughly the same. The data should be presented and compared with a statistical test to ensure that the baseline characteristics are similar. If they are not, then adjustments should be made using statistical techniques to ensure that bias from baseline differences did not interfere with the results.

Examples A study aimed to investigate whether selenium supplements prevented people with thyroid antibodies developing hypothyroidism [37]. There were several warning signs about this paper (retrospective design, small number of participants, low impact factor of journal), including significant differences in the baseline characteristics of the patient groups in age and TSH levels. The study claimed that selenium supplements were effective. A recent large randomised, blinded study has shown that although thyroid antibody levels reduce after selenium supplements, the development of hypothyroidism is not prevented [38].

Does the Study Have the 'Power' to Detect the Effects It Is Seeking?

Studying human beings is hard, not least because we differ so much from each other. But we also share a common biology, and all of us obey the rules of nature. So despite these individual variations, it is possible to tease out differences that may be related to specific factors, for example, lifestyle or exposure to a particular treatment. 'Power' is the ability of a study design to give a clear answer. Power depends on the number of subjects studied, the type of measurements we take and how certain we wish to be.

When designing a study, it is important to know in advance how many patients should be recruited and studied (we call this the 'sample size'), in order to have a good chance of answering the research question. As a general rule, the more the better, but that is too vague and rather unhelpful. Ideally one wishes to have sufficient numbers to be confident that what is observed represents a real phenomenon. Being 'confident' is one of the important parameters that are used to calculate the number of subjects needed. In biology, it is conventional and widely accepted that a convincing and appropriate level of confidence is 95% certainty.

Examples Consider that some people with hypothyroidism report that a particular nutritional supplement controls their hypothyroidism better than no supplement. If we wish to test this, we need to choose a measure of how well patients feel. ThyPRO is a well-designed and tested quality-of-life questionnaire designed for thyroid patients and would be a good choice [39]. Any measurement, if repeated, will show fluctuations. Measuring the weight of a kilo of potatoes multiple times will give you a slightly different reading around the average of 1 kg. This 'wobble' depends on how precise the scales are. If they are extremely good, the variation will be very small. In the case of ThyPRO, developing the questionnaire included such repeated measurements (called test-retest reliability) [40], and this is helpful in working out how many patients will be needed for such a study (we call this 'the sample size calculation').

The final bit of information in calculating the sample size is the difference we are looking for or 'effect size'. In other words, what difference in the ThyPRO score would we consider as being meaningful? Would a difference of 1% or 2% be enough to convince us that taking the supplement is worthwhile? Again, as part of the development of ThyPRO, researchers worked out the 'minimal important change' (MIC) [41], that is the minimum change in the ThyPRO score that patients perceive as important. It turns out that the MIC figure is about 10 (the ThyPRO scale ranges between 0 and 100). So now we have all the information for calculating how many subjects may be needed for the study. Doing the maths shows that about 200 patients will be required to get an answer to the original question of whether a nutritional supplement improves patients' quality of life, in order be 80% confident that such a study can provide a clear answer (is adequately 'powered').

Information about power calculations usually appears in the Methods section. The absence of power calculations is a signal of probable poor quality. A publication in 2017 showed that patients receiving combination treatment with levothyroxine and liothyronine who also had some genetic markers (of a transporter thyroid hormone gene and a deiodinase gene), preferred combination treatment [42]. The total number of patients studied was 45. No power calculation was performed. Four years later, the same authors wrote that studies on combination treatment previously published were not 'adequately powered' and that for such studies a sample size of over 300 subjects would be required [43].

Are the Statistical Tests Appropriate?

This is a challenging question for the non-expert and even academics can struggle with stats. But there are some obvious things that can be sought. If complex and obscure statistical tests are being used, the authors should explain why and provide references. The investigators should decide before the study commences what will be compared with what and with what statistical method.

Beware of comparisons being made between subgroups defined in retrospect (the jargon for this is called 'post-hoc analysis'). This is likely to introduce bias. Another trap is making multiple comparisons of several parameters between groups. The more the comparisons, the more likely that some will appear to be significant by chance. If such comparisons are made, there is a need to correct the calculations for the number of comparisons, and this should be stated; thus, look out for such a statement in the statistical methods section. Beware of studies claiming that they have unravelled important findings without stating the statistical tests used.

Examples One of the early studies on combination treatment of hypothyroidism with levothyroxine and liothyronine used 33 psychological tests [44], many of which were found to improve with combination treatment. Besides the fact that the study had too few patients (only 33), the authors also did not make appropriate corrections in the statistical calculations to account for the large number of psychological tests. Doing the statistics properly may have produced negative results. A much better-designed study of 697 hypothyroid patients found that combination with levothyroxine and liothyronine did not improve the quality of life compared to the placebo [45].

How Have the Authors Handled Missing Data?

It is almost inevitable that some data will be missing by the time of completion of any study. Researchers that care about eliminating bias due to missing data will have taken measures to address this problem. This is important because missing data can introduce errors. For instance, if a treatment causes side effects, participants who experience them may decide to come off the study prematurely, so the investigators are left with a subpopulation who happened to tolerate the treatment.

There are valid and statistically robust ways of ensuring that missing data do not bias the results, so information on how the authors handled missing data should be provided in the Methods section and the number of missing data should be reported and should be a small fraction of the total.

Are Early Stops Justified?

Some randomised controlled trials are terminated earlier than the study protocol dictates. There may be good reasons for that. If a treatment is associated with serious side effects, it would not be ethical to expose participants to the risk. On the other hand, if a life-saving treatment is clearly better than another, it would be unethical to allow a group of patients to continue on the inferior treatment. Sometimes a response to treatment (say at 3 months) may disappear at 6 months despite continuing the treatment. If the researchers decide to include the results only up to 3 months, the conclusions about the treatment may not be valid. The reasons for early stops should therefore be described in detail so that the reader can judge whether they were justified or not.

Are the Measurements Validated?

Nearly all scientific original publications include measuring something. It may be a laboratory test such as the serum free T3 level, exophthalmos (amount of protrusion of the eyeballs in patients with thyroid eye disease) or quality of life. It is important that these measurements do what they are supposed to. If the method for measuring free T3 is unreliable, the results may reflect the unreliability of the measurement more accurately than the actual true free T3 level.

The paper should provide information about validation and the performance of the measurements used and, if appropriate, cite relevant references. 'Validation' means making sure that what you measure is reliable. You can judge roughly the weight of a bag of potatoes by lifting it, but it will never be as good as a good set of properly calibrated scales. You can define how accurate the measurement is (or validate it) by repeating the measurements several times and using different weights. The absence of such information is not a good sign.

Is the Methodology Sufficiently Detailed for Replication?

The Methods section should provide enough detail for an independent team of investigators to repeat the study, if they so wished. It is the same principle as following a recipe. Without precise instructions about how to prepare a sumptuous dish, you will not be able to reproduce it and you will never know if the recipe's claim of how wonderful it tastes is actually true.

Are Conflicts of Interest Declared?

Most journals require that authors declare conflicts of interest. The absence of any statement on potential conflicts of interest should raise questions. Although declaring conflicts of interest does not eliminate such bias, at the very least it indicates that the authors and journal are mindful of the risks.

Is There Information About the Funding of the Study?

Studies funded by public sources usually are subjected to scrupulous review by the funding body before being supported. Studies supported by the pharmaceutical industry statistically are more prone to bias than those funded by the public sector [46].

Was There a Formal Process for Study Oversight?

Like school inspectors and business auditors, research should be conducted according to the rules of ethics and good practice. This is known as 'study oversight', and its absence may compromise quality [47] (note, however, that study oversight is a relatively recent concept and not applicable to studies performed more than 20–30 years ago).

Was the Study Registered?

Trial registration (ISRCTN registry, EU Clinical Trials Registry or ClinicalTrials.gov) is another component of good research practice and should be noted (note, however, that study registration is a relatively recent concept and not applicable to studies performed before 2005).

Was Ethical Approval Granted?

Ethical matters are important in research, and they are safeguarded by institutional frameworks. All research, particularly when it involves interventions, needs to be based on sound ethical grounds and to be in accordance with the Helsinki Declaration on human rights. All human and animal studies should include a statement on ethical approval and, if not applicable, should explain why.

Are the Results Reproducible?

On a cold November afternoon in the late 1970s, I found myself sitting in a seminar for final-year medical students led by Mike Rawlins. He was a Clinical Pharmacologist and after a 45-min discussion on medical research he concluded *'you need at least two independent studies pointing in the same direction to be confident that the results are reliable'*.

Our paths met several years later as colleagues. During one of the weekly Medical Grand Rounds at Freeman Hospital in Newcastle, he repeated what I had heard when I was his student.

Professor Sir Michael Rawlins was a fervent supporter of evidence-based medicine and chaired the National Institute for Health and Care Excellence from its foundation in 1999 for 14 years. If your search has led you to more than one paper showing similar findings, then 'Rawlin's law' will have been fulfilled. But such luxuries in medical research are still relatively rare.

For laboratory-based studies, the paper should include reproducibility data, that is, the experiments should be repeated and there should be consistency.

Laboratory reproducibility can have twists and turns as in the case of one of the most influential discoveries in the twentieth century. The Nobel laureate Cesar Milstein and his colleagues discovered 'monoclonal antibodies' in 1975. This was destined to revolutionise the treatment of cancer, autoimmune conditions like rheumatoid arthritis, thyroid eye disease and transplant rejection, to name a few of the beneficiaries of this amazing advance. He published his findings in the scientific journal *Nature* [48]. Although the experiments had been repeated dozens of times in his lab before the publication, suddenly they ceased to be reproducible. He and his co-workers tried hard to work out why, to no avail. The possibility that what they had observed was a laboratory error was beginning to dawn on them like a dark veil.

Milstein decided to do what every honest and self-respecting person should do. Accept that there may have been an error, retract his publication, eat humble pie, try to understand why it happened and start all over again [49]. Happily, his team defeated the laboratory gremlins and they were able to show that their results were real and reproducible.

In the thyroid field, examples of studies that produced positive results, which were subsequently impossible to replicate include a study in patients with Graves' disease claiming that administering levothyroxine together with anti-thyroid drugs was more effective than anti-thyroid drugs alone [50], a study claiming that the drug octreotide was effective in patients with thyroid eye disease [19], and a study claiming that combination treatment with levothyroxine and liothyronine led to better symptom control than levothyroxine alone [44].

Putting It All Together

If you have identified a red flag (paper has NOT been peer reviewed), you can safely reject it as highly likely to be unreliable (Fig. 5.1). If you have picked up a green flag (paper supported by an independent study with similar results,

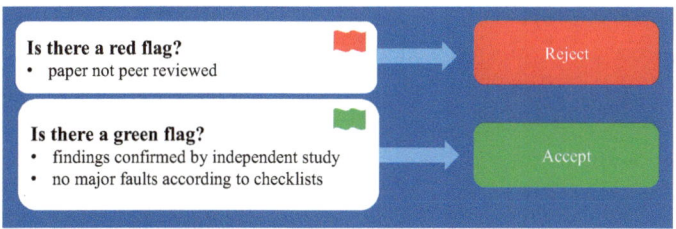

Fig. 5.1 Red and green flags for the quality of publications

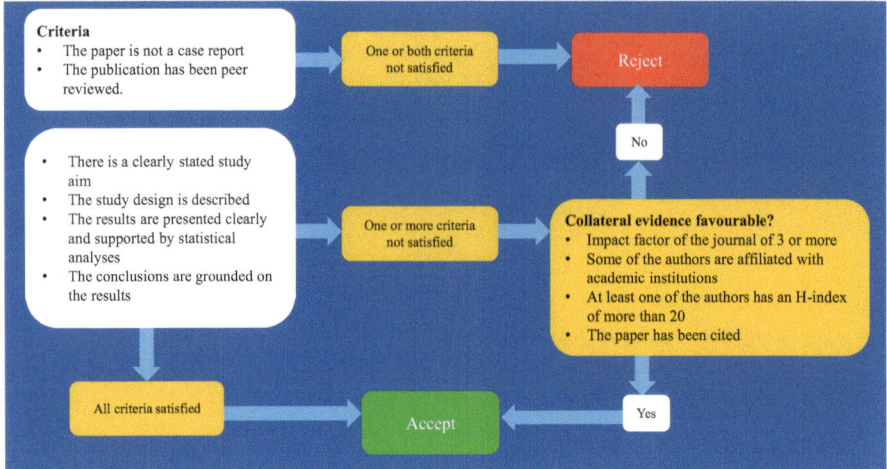

Fig. 5.2 Summary of simple appraisal checklist for the quality of publications

there are no other papers contradicting the evidence and not a litany of other faults picked up by the checklists), then the paper probably deserves your trust and attention.

If all you have to go by is the Simple Checklist (Fig. 5.2) and if you have found no faults in the bullet points, and the Collateral evidence is favourable (impact factor of the journal of three or more, at least some of the authors are affiliated with academic institutions, at least one of the authors has an H-index of more than 20), then you can conclude that the paper may be valid, but this is a blunt instrument, and all but the poorest papers will have passed this test.

If you have had the opportunity and the courage to follow the Advanced Appraisal Checklist (Fig. 5.3), then you can use a scoring system that you can feed the labours of your appraisal, which will give you an idea of the quality of the paper that you have appraised. Consider the bullet points in the Advanced Appraisal Checklist. Ignore those items that are not applicable (study registration may not be relevant because the paper was published before 2005 when it was not a requirement, or you feel unable to judge whether the statistics were appropriate). For the rest of the items in the Advance Checklist, you can place a tick or a cross depending on whether the criterion described is satisfied or not. Sum up all the ticks and work out the percentage ([ticks/ticks + crosses] × 100). You will end up with a figure between 0 and 100%. The closer to the top the of the scale, the more likely that the publication is of good quality and the reverse. Validated methods for pursuing the same are available (see below under 'Further reading'), but they are complex, are intended for experts and are very hard to follow for most lay people.

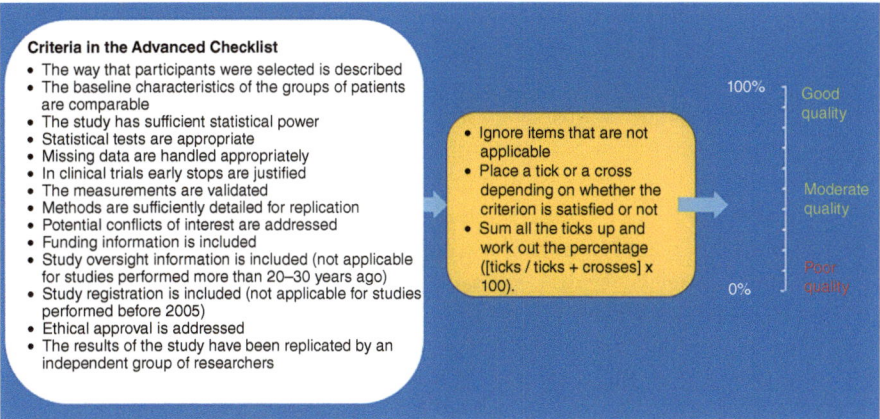

Criteria in the Advanced Checklist
- The way that participants were selected is described
- The baseline characteristics of the groups of patients are comparable
- The study has sufficient statistical power
- Statistical tests are appropriate
- Missing data are handled appropriately
- In clinical trials early stops are justified
- The measurements are validated
- Methods are sufficiently detailed for replication
- Potential conflicts of interest are addressed
- Funding information is included
- Study oversight information is included (not applicable for studies performed more than 20–30 years ago)
- Study registration is included (not applicable for studies performed before 2005)
- Ethical approval is addressed
- The results of the study have been replicated by an independent group of researchers

- Ignore items that are not applicable
- Place a tick or a cross depending on whether the criterion is satisfied or not
- Sum all the ticks up and work out the percentage ([ticks / ticks + crosses] x 100).

100% — Good quality

Moderate quality

0% — Poor quality

Fig. 5.3 Summary of advanced appraisal checklist for the quality of publications

Appraising the evidence is not simple. Scrutinising papers using the criteria outlined above will pick up faults in many publications. This should not lead to automatic rejection, but the more problems identified the more concerned you should be about its worth. Appraising the evidence is not black and white, judgement improves with experience and there is always a possibility that the appraiser may get it wrong.

Further Reading

There is a large body of literature about 'critical appraisal' of medical evidence. For readers wishing to expand their knowledge on the subject, an excellent document by Amanda Burls of Oxford University is freely available on the Internet and is worth reading [51]. The website 'Science or not?' [52] is also a valuable source of information on how to weigh up scientific evidence. The DISCERN tool [53] offers guidance about judging the quality of a publication about treatments. There are more complex, formalised ways of assessing the quality of medical publications [54], including CASP [55] and the Jadad score [56].

References

1. BTAThyroidCancerGuidelines2002. Guidelines for the management of thyroid cancer in adults; 2002.
2. BTAThyroidCancerGuidelines2007. Guidelines for the management of thyroid cancer. Royal College of Physicians; 2007.

3. Perros P, Boelaert K, Colley S, et al. Guidelines for the management of thyroid cancer. Clin Endocrinol (Oxf). 2014;81(Suppl 1):1–122. https://doi.org/10.1111/cen.12515.

4. NICEThyroidCancer. https://www.nice.org.uk/guidance/ng230.

5. Braverman LE, Ingbar SH, Sterling K. Conversion of thyroxine (T4) to triiodothyronine (T3) in athyreotic human subjects. J Clin Invest. 1970;49(5):855–64. https://doi.org/10.1172/JCI106304.

6. Watson JD, Crick FH. Molecular structure of nucleic acids; a structure for deoxyribose nucleic acid. Nature. 1953;171(4356):737–8. https://doi.org/10.1038/171737a0.

7. Engel FL. An unusual case of malignant exophthalmos and postoperative hypothyroidism complicating Graves' disease. J Clin Endocrinol Metab. 1953;13(9):1132–9. https://doi.org/10.1210/jcem-13-9-1132.

8. Wakefield AJ, Murch SH, Anthony A, et al. Ileal-lymphoid-nodular hyperplasia, non-specific colitis, and pervasive developmental disorder in children. Lancet. 1998;351(9103):637–41. https://doi.org/10.1016/s0140-6736(97)11096-0.

9. Scopus. https://www.scopus.com/.

10. PubMed. https://pubmed.ncbi.nlm.nih.gov/help/#how-do-i-search-pubmed.

11. WebofScience. https://clarivate.com/webofsciencegroup/solutions/web-of-science/.

12. Pollack L. Treating thyroid dysfunction. Homeopathy In Pract. 2007;1000:46.

13. Tang Y, Xing Y, Lin MT, Zhang J, Jia J. Hashimoto's encephalopathy cases: Chinese experience. BMC Neurol. 2012;12:60. https://doi.org/10.1186/1471-2377-12-60.

14. Gussekloo J, van Exel E, de Craen AJ, Meinders AE, Frolich M, Westendorp RG. Thyroid status, disability and cognitive function, and survival in old age. JAMA. 2004;292(21):2591–9. https://doi.org/10.1001/jama.292.21.2591.

15. Avramenko N, Barkovskiy D, Postolenko V. Ozone therapy of the adenomyosis at women with sterility and hypothyroidism. ScienceRise Med Sci. 2017;20(4):20–4.

16. Walsh JP, Ward LC, Burke V, et al. Small changes in thyroxine dosage do not produce measurable changes in hypothyroid symptoms, well-being, or quality of life: results of a double-blind, randomized clinical trial. J Clin Endocrinol Metab. 2006;91(7):2624–30. https://doi.org/10.1210/jc.2006-0099.

17. Joshi R, Kumar P, et al. Clinical evaluation of Agnimandhya virechana yoga in the management of hypothyroidism. Int J Ayurveda Pharma Res. 2019;7(8):29–34.

18. Massolt ET, van der Windt M, Korevaar TI, et al. Thyroid hormone and its metabolites in relation to quality of life in patients treated for differentiated thyroid cancer. Clin Endocrinol (Oxf). 2016;85(5):781–8. https://doi.org/10.1111/cen.13101.

19. Krassas GE, Dumas A, Pontikides N, Kaltsas T. Somatostatin receptor scintigraphy and octreotide treatment in patients with thyroid eye disease. Clin Endocrinol (Oxf). 1995;42(6):571–80. https://doi.org/10.1111/j.1365-2265.1995.tb02682.x.

20. Dickinson AJ, Vaidya B, Miller M, et al. Double-blind, placebo-controlled trial of octreotide long-acting repeatable (LAR) in thyroid-associated ophthalmopathy. J Clin Endocrinol Metab. 2004;89(12):5910–5. https://doi.org/10.1210/jc.2004-0697.
21. Stan MN, Garrity JA, Bradley EA, et al. Randomized, double-blind, placebo-controlled trial of long-acting release octreotide for treatment of Graves' ophthalmopathy. J Clin Endocrinol Metab. 2006;91(12):4817–24. https://doi.org/10.1210/jc.2006-1105.
22. Wemeau JL, Caron P, Beckers A, et al. Octreotide (long-acting release formulation) treatment in patients with Graves' orbitopathy: clinical results of a four-month, randomized, placebo-controlled, double-blind study. J Clin Endocrinol Metab. 2005;90(2):841–8. https://doi.org/10.1210/jc.2004-1334.
23. Lowe JC. Thyroid status of 38 fibromyalgia patients: implications for the etiology of fibromyalgia. Clin Bull Myofascial Ther. 1996;10(2):47–64.
24. Lowe JC, Garrison RL, et al. Effectiveness and safety of T3 (triiodothyronine) therapy for euthyroid fibromyalgia: a double-blind placebo-controlled response-driven crossover study. Clin Bull Myofascial Ther. 1996;2(2–3):31–57.
25. Lowe JC. Results of an open trial of T3 therapy with 77 euthyroid female fibromyalgia patients. Clin Bull Myofascial Ther. 1996;2(1):35–7.
26. Macfarlane GJ, Kronisch C, Dean LE, et al. EULAR revised recommendations for the management of fibromyalgia. Ann Rheum Dis. 2017;76(2):318–28. https://doi.org/10.1136/annrheumdis-2016-209724.
27. Skinner GRB, Holmes D, et al. Clinical response to thyroxine sodium in clinically hypothyroid but biochemically euthyroid patients. J Nutr Environ Med. 2000;10(2):115–24.
28. Pollock MA, Sturrock A, Marshall K, et al. Thyroxine treatment in patients with symptoms of hypothyroidism but thyroid function tests within the reference range: randomised double blind placebo controlled crossover trial. BMJ. 2001;323(7318):891–5. https://doi.org/10.1136/bmj.323.7318.891.
29. Hirsch JE. An index to quantify an individual's scientific research output. Proc Natl Acad Sci U S A. 2005;102(46):16569–72. https://doi.org/10.1073/pnas.0507655102.
30. Cohen Y, Xing M, Mambo E, et al. BRAF mutation in papillary thyroid carcinoma. J Natl Cancer Inst. 2003;95(8):625–7. https://doi.org/10.1093/jnci/95.8.625.
31. Subbiah V, Kreitman RJ, Wainberg ZA, et al. Dabrafenib and Trametinib treatment in patients with locally advanced or metastatic BRAF V600-mutant anaplastic thyroid cancer. J Clin Oncol. 2018;36(1):7–13. https://doi.org/10.1200/JCO.2017.73.6785.
32. Saravanan P, Chau WF, Roberts N, Vedhara K, Greenwood R, Dayan CM. Psychological well-being in patients on 'adequate' doses of l-thyroxine: results of a large, controlled community-based questionnaire study. Clin Endocrinol (Oxf). 2002;57(5):577–85. https://doi.org/10.1046/j.1365-2265.2002.01654.x.

33. Taylor PN, Iqbal A, Minassian C, et al. Falling threshold for treatment of border-line elevated thyrotropin levels-balancing benefits and risks: evidence from a large community-based study. JAMA Intern Med. 2014;174(1):32–9. https://doi.org/10.1001/jamainternmed.2013.11312.
34. Carle A, Karmisholt JS, Knudsen N, et al. Does subclinical hypothyroidism add any symptoms? Evidence from a Danish population-based study. Am J Med. 2021;134(9):1115–1126.e1. https://doi.org/10.1016/j.amjmed.2021.03.009.
35. Brito JP, Ross JS, El Kawkgi OM, et al. Levothyroxine use in the United States, 2008-2018. JAMA Intern Med. 2021;181(10):1402–5. https://doi.org/10.1001/jamainternmed.2021.2686.
36. Burgos N, Toloza FJK, Singh Ospina NM, et al. Clinical outcomes after discontinuation of thyroid hormone replacement: a systematic review and meta-analysis. Thyroid. 2021;31(5):740–51. https://doi.org/10.1089/thy.2020.0679.
37. Pace C, Tumino D, Russo M, et al. Role of selenium and myo-inositol supplementation on autoimmune thyroiditis progression. Endocr J. 2020;67(11):1093–8. https://doi.org/10.1507/endocrj.EJ20-0062.
38. Larsen C, Winther KH, Cramon PK, Rasmussen AK, Feldt-Rasmusssen U, Knudsen NJ, Bjorner JB, Schomburg L, Demircan K, Chillon TS, Gram J, Hansen SG, Brandt F, Nygaard B, Watt T, Hegedus L, Bonnema SJ. Selenium supplementation and placebo are equally effective in improving quality of life in patients with hypothyroidism. Eur Thyroid J. 2024;13(1):e230175. https://doi.org/10.1530/ETJ-23-0175.
39. Watt T, Bjorner JB, Groenvold M, et al. Development of a short version of the thyroid-related patient-reported outcome ThyPRO. Thyroid. 2015;25(10):1069–79. https://doi.org/10.1089/thy.2015.0209.
40. Watt T, Hegedus L, Groenvold M, et al. Validity and reliability of the novel thyroid-specific quality of life questionnaire, ThyPRO. Eur J Endocrinol. 2010;162(1):161–7. https://doi.org/10.1530/EJE-09-0521.
41. Nordqvist SF, Boesen VB, Rasmussen AK, et al. Determining minimal important change for the thyroid-related quality of life questionnaire ThyPRO. Endocr Connect. 2021;10(3):316–24. https://doi.org/10.1530/EC-21-0026.
42. Carle A, Faber J, Steffensen R, Laurberg P, Nygaard B. Hypothyroid patients encoding combined MCT10 and DIO2 gene polymorphisms may prefer L-T3 + L-T4 combination treatment—data using a blind, randomized, clinical study. Eur Thyroid J. 2017;6(3):143–51. https://doi.org/10.1159/000469709.
43. Jonklaas JBA, Cappola AR, Celi FS, Fliers E, Heuer H, McAninch EA, Moeller LC, Nygaard B, Sawka AM, Watt T, Dayan CM. Evidence-based use of levothyroxine/liothyronine combinations in treating hypothyroidism: a consensus document. Eur Thyroid J. 2021;31:156–82.
44. Bunevicius R, Kazanavicius G, Zalinkevicius R, Prange AJ Jr. Effects of thyroxine as compared with thyroxine plus triiodothyronine in patients with hypothyroidism. N Engl J Med. 1999;340(6):424–9. https://doi.org/10.1056/NEJM199902113400603.

45. Saravanan P, Simmons DJ, Greenwood R, Peters TJ, Dayan CM. Partial substitution of thyroxine (T4) with tri-iodothyronine in patients on T4 replacement therapy: results of a large community-based randomized controlled trial. J Clin Endocrinol Metab. 2005;90(2):805–12. https://doi.org/10.1210/jc.2004-1672.
46. Lexchin J. Sponsorship bias in clinical research. Int J Risk Saf Med. 2012;24(4):233–42. https://doi.org/10.3233/JRS-2012-0574.
47. Umscheid CA, Margolis DJ, Grossman CE. Key concepts of clinical trials: a narrative review. Postgrad Med. 2011;123(5):194–204. https://doi.org/10.3810/pgm.2011.09.2475.
48. Kohler G, Milstein C. Continuous cultures of fused cells secreting antibody of predefined specificity. Nature. 1975;256(5517):495–7. https://doi.org/10.1038/256495a0.
49. Milstein C. https://biolegend.com/ja-jp/blog/discovery-series-hybridomas.
50. Hashizume K, Ichikawa K, Sakurai A, et al. Administration of thyroxine in treated Graves' disease. Effects on the level of antibodies to thyroid-stimulating hormone receptors and on the risk of recurrence of hyperthyroidism. N Engl J Med. 1991;324(14):947–53. https://doi.org/10.1056/NEJM199104043241403.
51. WhatIsCriticalAppraisal? http://www.bandolier.org.uk/painres/download/whatis/What_is_critical_appraisal.pdf.
52. ScienceOrNot? https://scienceornot.net/.
53. DISCERNtool. http://www.discern.org.uk/about.php.
54. Pastorino R, Milovanovic S, Stojanovic J, Efremov L, Amore R, Boccia S. Quality assessment of studies published in open access and subscription journals: results of a systematic evaluation. PLoS One. 2016;11(5):e0154217. https://doi.org/10.1371/journal.pone.0154217.
55. CASP. https://casp-uk.net/.
56. Jadad AR, Moore RA, Carroll D, et al. Assessing the quality of reports of randomized clinical trials: is blinding necessary? Control Clin Trials. 1996;17(1):1–12. https://doi.org/10.1016/0197-2456(95)00134-4.

6

Interpreting the Evidence

'The real quandary about correlations and associations is whether there is a cause-and-effect relationship'.

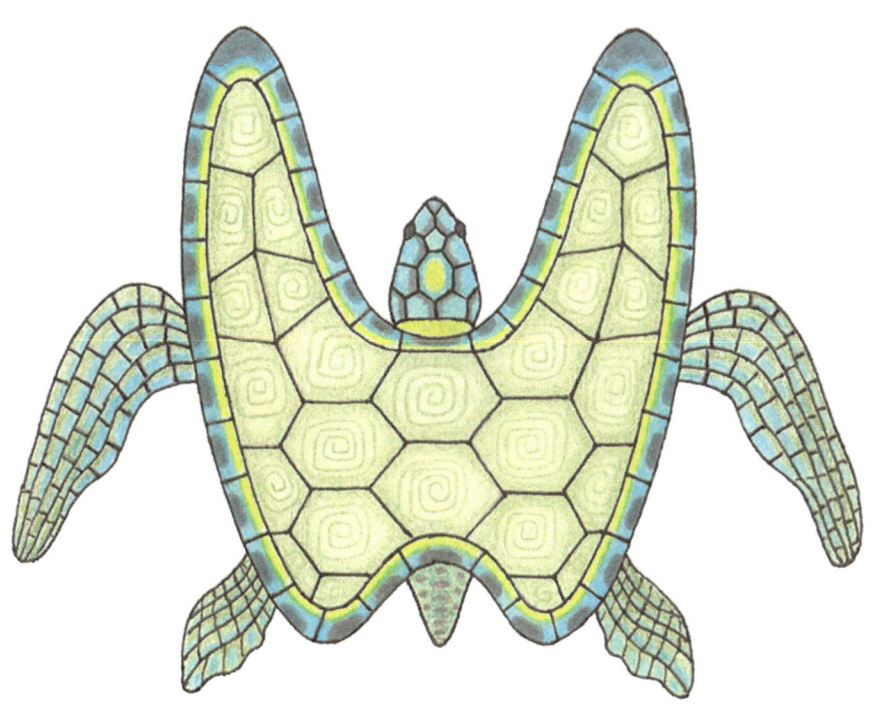

An Early South Glasgow Lesson

Halfway through my second year after qualifying as a doctor, I took up a post as Senior House Officer at one of Glasgow's hospitals. I was enamoured by the old Victorian building, its ambience, the colleagues and the patients. The clientele was a mix of social backgrounds, some utterly impoverished and others (residents of leafy Shawlands) very well-heeled.

The patient in question was of the latter kind, well dressed, articulate and terribly worried. She listed numerous symptoms and complaints. After taking a thorough history and performing a detailed examination, I found nothing out of order. I requested some blood tests. They all came back normal. I wrote a lengthy letter to her family doctor describing my findings. A few weeks later, I was summoned by my consultant. He was about to review the patient in his clinic and had read my notes and letter. He asked me if I remembered the case, which I did, and in a somewhat irritated tone asked, *do you think her symptoms are functional or organic?* In other words, did this patient have an identifiable underlying disease, or were the symptoms largely psychological? It suddenly dawned on me that having diligently collected all the evidence I could generate and having documented it in detail in the patient's record, I failed to complete the most important part of my assessment. To interpret the evidence and give it some form of rational meaning by formulating an opinion. This same concept applies to published medical evidence.

Turtles have a thyroid gland that looks more like a beetle rather than a butterfly. Tri-iodothyronine (T3) is said to play an important role in determining the sex of the turtle offspring, but this claim has not been confirmed by another independents study [1]. *Although an interesting story, the jury is still out about the true role of T3 in turtle sex determination.*

Interpreting the evidence is the most difficult part of getting to the truth and hardest to break down into small mouthfuls. It is because prior knowledge, both specialised and broad about the topic, experience, a sixth sense for what is plausible and what is 'too good to be true', are all required. So, initial attempts to interpret the evidence will probably fail, but with experience, expanding knowledge and perseverance, it will become easier to pass ultimate judgment.

Tables, Figures and Supplements

The section of the paper that the interpretation is based on is the 'Results', the real meat of the report. It consists of the text, tables, figures and often supplementary material. The authors will have selected the findings that they wish to highlight in tables and particularly in figures. The data will have been analysed statistically, and significant differences and findings will be highlighted.

A good start is to look at the tables and figures and try to work out for yourself what they mean. Is one treatment better than another? Does a participant characteristic (e.g. smoking) link with another (e.g. development of thyroid eye disease). Does looking at the tables and figures help to build up a narrative that derives from the data and makes sense? Can you see any obvious holes in the presentation of the results? Reading the text in the Results section will provide additional nuance and context, which will help you understand the data.

Once you have digested the results, read the discussion section and see how much agreement there is between what you think the results mean compared to the authors. They are bound to differ, but does the discussion convince you of the authors' conclusions? In many papers (at least those published in the past decade), the authors refer to the limitations of their study and how they have addressed them. Does that account seem fair and persuasive? Interventional studies that aim to evaluate a treatment such as a drug or a procedure should report both 'efficacy' (how effective the treatment) as well as side effects, and the verdict should be a balanced opinion that takes all aspects of the intervention into consideration.

Stats, Again…

My relationship with stats has been love and hate over the years and to be frank more hate than love. I blame my non-mathematical brain and an early negative experience with a senior statistician. I had just entered the realm of research and needed some advice on how to handle the data I had gathered on a study of a drug called azathioprine in patients with thyroid eye disease [2]. The senior statistician firstly gave me a severe dressing down for not seeking advice before starting the data collection, then rubbished what I had done and sent me packing.

I have since met and collaborated with several statisticians who have been extremely helpful, professional and kind, so my faith has been restored, but traces of the trauma remain and my heart rate accelerates when I meet one. They speak to me in Statish, I reply in Thyrish and we get along fine.

Unfortunately, I need to introduce some Statish terms which may sound like the plot from an Alfred Hitchcock movie ('deviation', 'mean', 'risk'). Statistics are used to describe data, compare groups of data and examine relationships between groups to determine if differences are likely to be real or random. Here I cover some of the common statistical concepts. You will encounter many more in your searches, which would be impossible to describe in this book, and you may have to make additional efforts to discover what they mean.

Descriptive Stats

Means, Medians, Standard Deviations, Ranges, Confidence Intervals, Percentages

The age of participants or size of a thyroid nodule are called 'continuous' data because there are no gaps, so one can be exactly 25.0 years old on their birthday or 25.35 or anywhere in between; in contrast your child can either be in year 5 or 6, which is 'categorical' data. Data like age are typically summarised in publications by quoting the average (a measure of the centre of the data, such as 'mean', 'median' and 'mode'), 'standard deviation' (a measure of the spread of the data), 95% 'confidence intervals' (a spread within which we expect the average to be) and 'range' (smallest to largest measurement). These parameters provide a descriptive summary of the data.

It is important that we use both the average and the scatter around it when we think about data. Suppose that a weather forecaster predicts that there is 'a 35% chance of rain' for tomorrow. Now imagine that they forecast that there is '10–60% chance of rain'. Does that change your mind about taking an umbrella when you go out? And what if they narrow it to '30–40% chance of rain'? Most of us are likely to take the 30–40% prediction more seriously than the 10–60%, because 30–40% seems more precise, although the average is the same.

The 95% confidence interval consists of two numbers, a low and a high limit. It tells us that we can be 95% certain that the average will lie within the two numbers. The standard deviation is also a measure of spread. In a set of data, 95% will be within two standard deviations from the average. The wider the confidence intervals and the higher the standard deviation (in comparison to the mean), the more aware you should be about the limitations of the estimate.

The number of observations (or measurements) we make has a major influence on the confidence intervals and on judging whether two groups that are being compared are different from each other. Here is an example. A long time ago, a colleague was involved in a study that aimed to investigate whether the size of the thyroid gland was greater in pregnant compared with non-pregnant women. It was known that sometimes pregnant women developed a goitre, but the documentation was based on small numbers and used unreliable methods for measuring the thyroid size. Interestingly, it is said that ancient Egyptians used to tie a reed around the neck of young women, and when the reed snapped, this early pregnancy test was considered positive [3].

In my colleague's study, ultrasound was used to measure the size of the thyroid gland of pregnant women in the middle of the second trimester. The scan was repeated one year after childbirth. As you can imagine it took a long time to collect the data. My impatient colleague started to look at the measurements when she had collected only six sets of data (Fig. 6.1).

The confidence intervals were wide, and eyeballing the results, there seemed to be little difference between the measurements during pregnancy and afterwards. Frankly, she was quite disappointed.

Six months later, she had 12 sets of data and she looked at them again. The confidence intervals had narrowed as the number of dots increased and things were looking up. It was becoming apparent that there may be a difference in the size of the thyroid, as expected: larger in the middle of pregnancy and smaller a year later (Fig. 6.2).

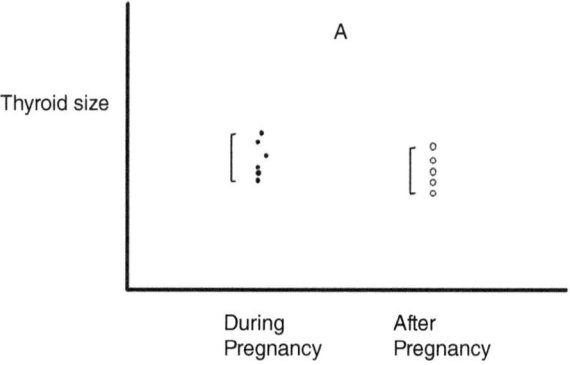

Fig. 6.1 Early results. The brackets show the confidence intervals

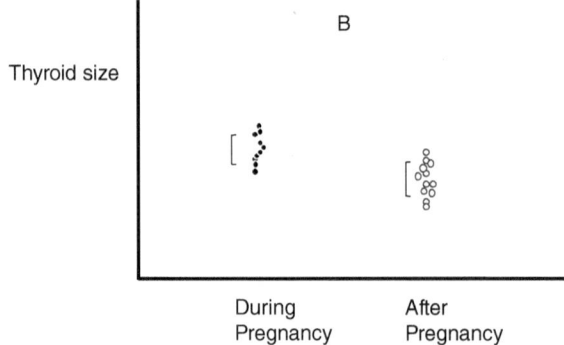

Fig. 6.2 Results 6 months later. The brackets show confidence intervals

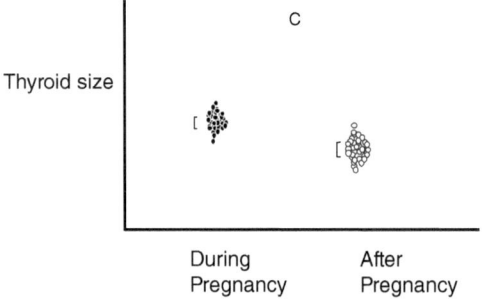

Fig. 6.3 Results at the end of the study. The brackets show confidence intervals

A year later she had accumulated a stunning 36 sets of measurements before and after childbirth (Fig. 6.3). The confidence intervals had narrowed further as more data had been added, the averages of two sets of dots had drifted apart and the 95% confidence intervals no longer overlapped. It looked like pregnancy was indeed associated with a larger-sized thyroid gland compared to a year after childbirth. My colleague was chuffed.

The irony is that had she discovered that there was no difference in the size of the thyroid during compared to after pregnancy, the result would have been just as important and scientifically valid. But you will remember from Chap. 3, we like positive results more than negative, and negative findings are more difficult to publish than positive.

The spread (or distribution) of data can tell us a lot, and this cannot be emphasised enough. Look at this map (Fig. 6.4). The black dots represent the place of residence of cholera victims in a 1854 outbreak in London. At the

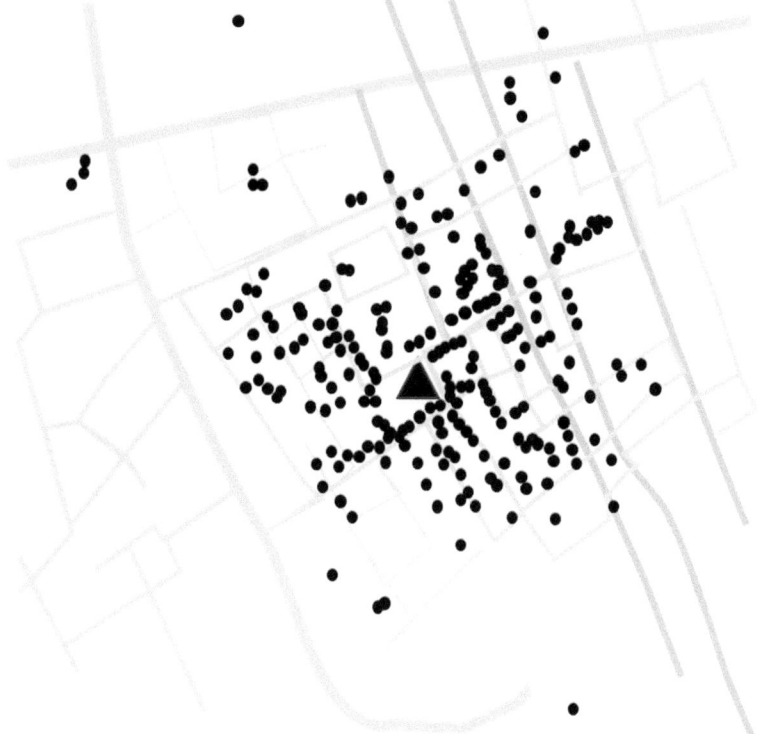

Fig. 6.4 Deaths from cholera in the 1854 London outbreak. The black dots show the place of residence of victims of cholera. The pump that provided drinking water is shown as a triangle (redrawn from https://en.wikipedia.org/wiki/File:Snow-cholera-map-1.jpg)

centre of the map was a water pump where local people got their drinking water. If one plots the number of deaths due to cholera against distance from the pump and places them into groups (0–10 yards, 11–19 yards, 20–29 yards etc.), then what emerges is a distribution curve (the negative numbers represent distance to the left, and the positive numbers to the right of an imaginary perpendicular line that crosses the pump on the map). The peak was the hotspot of cholera deaths and corresponded to where the water pump was situated (Fig. 6.5).

It is believed that it was exactly this relationship between deaths from cholera and where people lived in relation to the contaminated water pump that enabled John Snow to solve the puzzle (although the famous map was constructed after the epidemic).

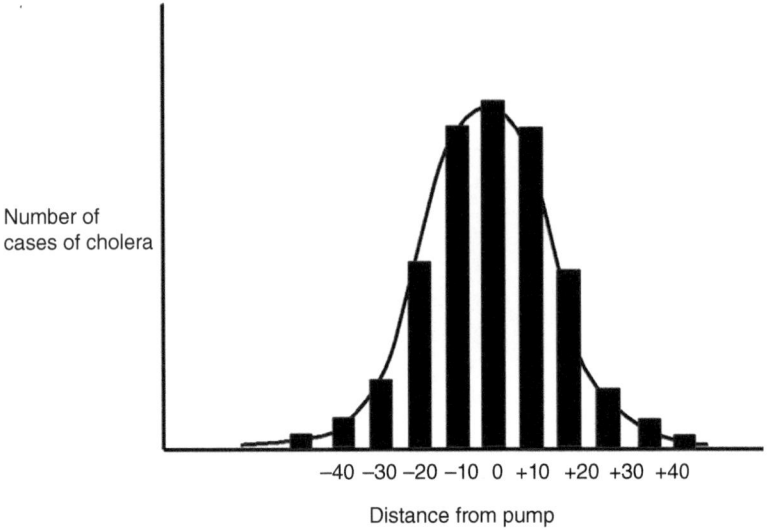

Fig. 6.5 Distribution of cases of cholera according to the distance of place of residence from the pump

John Snow is considered the founder of Public Health. He was born in York, educated in Newcastle upon Tyne and practiced as physician in London. He was interested in cholera and studied the 1854 outbreak in detail [4]. And here is a great part of the story. Finding the cause is, of course, important, but useless if you cannot find a solution. We know that carbon emissions are a major cause of climate change, but reversing it has turned out to be an enormously complicated and difficult task, and it is uncertain whether it can be fixed. In the case of the cholera outbreak, the solution was to remove the handle off the pump, thus disabling it and providing an alternative source of water: simple, radical and 100% effective.

Another example of how the distribution of data is used, which can affect people being investigated and treated for thyroid disease, relates to thyroid blood tests. If we consider the levels of TSH in the bloodstream of people who have no personal or family history of thyroid problems and are otherwise healthy, the distribution looks like Fig. 6.6 [5]. You will notice that it is not entirely symmetrical, and there is a bit of a tail to the right (shaded part of Fig. 6.6). On the basis of this information, it was suggested that the normal range for serum TSH should be between 0.45 and 4.12 mU/L.

It turned out that a significant number of subjects included in the data had positive thyroid antibodies, therefore may not have been 'normal'. Removing such patients resulted in some shift of the tail towards the left and the

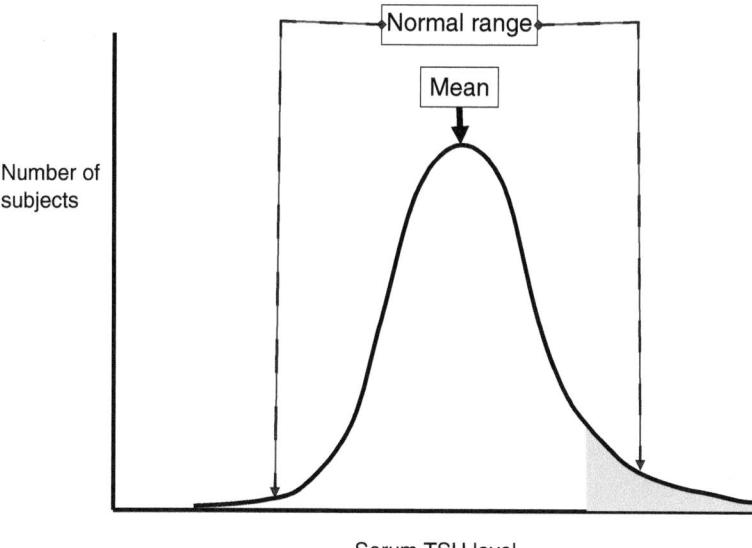

Fig. 6.6   Distribution of serum TSH in normal subjects

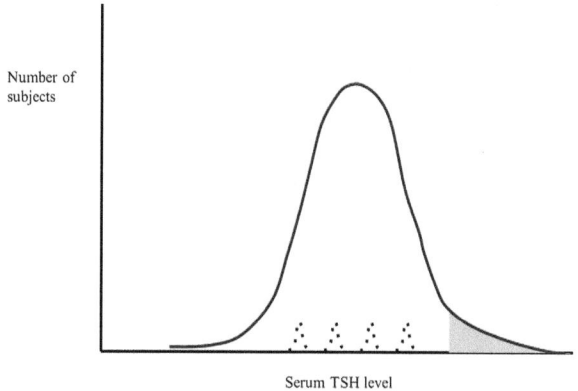

Fig. 6.7   Distribution of serum TSH in normal subjects after excluding people with positive thyroid antibodies. In addition, the interrupted lines show the distribution of serum TSH levels of four normal subjects measured several times over a year for each subject

suggestion that the upper limit of normal should be lowered to 2.5 mU/L [6]. However, the curve was still skewed to the right, though less so than before (Fig. 6.7).

There are other population characteristics that push the right-hand side of the curve outwards, like obesity, old age and ethnicity [7]. And it gets more complicated, because if one considers individual healthy subjects and measures their TSH on multiple occasions over time, the distribution curves for each person are pretty narrow, but differ from each other, although broadly within the 'normal range' (Fig. 6.7) [8].

The definition of the normal range for TSH and other thyroid blood tests has been debated intently and continues to be controversial, although a broad range such as in 0.45 and 4.12 mU/L is generally accepted by most experts [7]. An alternative way to trying to define the normal range is in the context of what happens to long-term health. This is explored further in Part III.

As already mentioned, data can also be 'categorical', where there are groups or 'categories' within the data. A two-category example would be a study investigating the effect of a cancer treatment. The patient outcome of mortality has two categories: 'alive' or 'deceased'. A common way of summarising categorical data is to use percentages or frequencies, for example, a UK study found that mortality figures from thyroid cancer at 10 years after diagnosis were 0% for stage I, 3.1% for stage II, 28.6% for stage III and 30% for stage IV [9] ('stage' is a measure of how advanced the cancer was at the time of diagnosis).

Statistical Significance

While there are some types of research where statistical analyses are not meaningful (called 'qualitative', e.g. based on interviews with patients or carers), the vast majority of studies include statistical calculations that tell us whether differences revealed by comparisons are 'significant'.

The way statisticians approach medical research is with apparent negativity. Instead of being bouncy, optimistic and hopeful, they do the exact opposite. Considering a study of a treatment that promises to lower thyroid antibodies and hopefully prevent autoimmune thyroid disease is better than no treatment. Statisticians tell us that we should assume that it will make no difference. In fact worse than that, they argue that any difference between treatment and no treatment demonstrated by their hard-working research colleagues who sweat it out on the coalface may be due to chance alone. They call this bad-tempered attitude, the 'null hypothesis'.

Then, using sorcery they work the data in their statistical cauldron and come up with a P value. 'P' stands for probability. The lower the P value, the more likely the statistician is wrong and the more joyful is the rest of the world. The cut-off for the P value being 'significant' (created arbitrarily by one of their lot and imposed on the rest of humanity) is 0.05, or 5%.

Now that my pent-up emotions due to my PTSD (post-traumatic *statistical disorder*) have been released, I can deal with this a little more rationally and concede that I have been unfair to statisticians. In fact the null hypothesis is what we tend to do when we think with Kahneman's System Two, that is, using our rational and just self. It is the same as approaching unexplained phenomena from a 'devil's advocate' perspective, applying the principle of 'innocent until proven guilty', 'Cromwell's rule' or Popper's 'black swan' argument. More often than not, the path in our quest for knowledge and truth forces us to have to face and reject what is false, rather than find and confirm what is true. A *P*-value of <0.05 or less tells us that the odds that a difference found between two or more sets of data has arisen by chance and is less than 5%. By convention we interpret this as being statistically significant and we feel reasonably confident that if we repeat the study our findings will be similar.

Another type of statistical analysis relates to 'correlations' or 'associations'. A correlation is a relationship between variables so that when one increases the other also alters proportionately, by increasing (positive correlation) or decreasing (negative correlation). An 'association' implies that knowing about one parameter also tells us about another. For instance, if a patient has a diagnosis of Hashimoto's thyroiditis, the likelihood is that she is female because many studies have shown that approximately 90% of patients with Hashimoto's thyroiditis are women. We can therefore posit that there is an association between Hashimoto's thyroiditis and gender.

In everyday life, there are correlations everywhere around us and we make simple and important decisions based on them. For example, we avoid (if we can) driving in the rush hour because there is a correlation between early morning and late afternoon times and how long it takes to get to our destination, and the closer we get to the rush hour, the longer we spend in our car fantasising about growing wings. In thyroid diseases, numerous associations have been found, for example, between hypothyroidism and other autoimmune diseases (like coeliac disease) [10], psychiatric illness [11], female sex [12] and iodine status [13].

The real quandary about correlations and associations is whether there is a cause-and-effect relationship (remember the cockerel's crow?). Observational studies are generally not designed to unravel causation, but the chances of a causal relationship are increased if some conditions are met, based on the 'Bradford-Hill criteria' named after those that invented them, some) [14].

Bradford-Hill Criteria for Causation
- There is a 'dose-response' relationship between the parameters.
- The presence of a biologically plausible mechanism for the relationship is causal.
- The relationship between the parameters is strong.
- The observations are reproducible.
- A specific population is affected by a specific disease in the absence of other explanations.
- The effect occurs after the exposure.
- The observations in a population are supported by laboratory evidence.

A good example is the relationship between smoking and thyroid eye disease. The link between the two has been noted in many studies [15]. Furthermore, the risk of thyroid eye disease is greater than larger the number of cigarettes smoked per day ('dose-response' relationship), smoking affects the immune system and encourages inflammation (biologically plausible mechanism) and smokers are three times more likely to suffer from thyroid eye disease (the relationship is strong) [16]. The link therefore between smoking and thyroid eye disease is likely causal, although the evidence is indirect and comes from cross-sectional studies.

Correlations relating to the thyroid include the continuing rise in new cases of thyroid cancer with time [17], a negative correlation between the serum level of TSH and free T4 in subjects with untreated hypothyroidism or hyperthyroidism [18] and a positive correlation between severity of thyroid eye disease and age [19] (Fig. 6.8).

The strength of a correlation is represented as the 'correlation coefficient'. This tells us how close the points are between the variables we are interested in, to a straight line. The correlation coefficient (called 'r') is equal to 1 (perfect) when all the dots fall on the straight line (Fig. 6.9a). This is extremely rare, and usually an r of say 0.8 is respectable (Fig. 6.9b). When there is no correlation and the dots are random, r equals 0 (Fig. 6.9c). If the correlation is negative, then r has a negative value (Fig. 6.9d).

The examples given above apply to a particular type of 'linear' correlation called 'Pearson's' for continuous variables. Other types of correlations exist for different kinds of data.

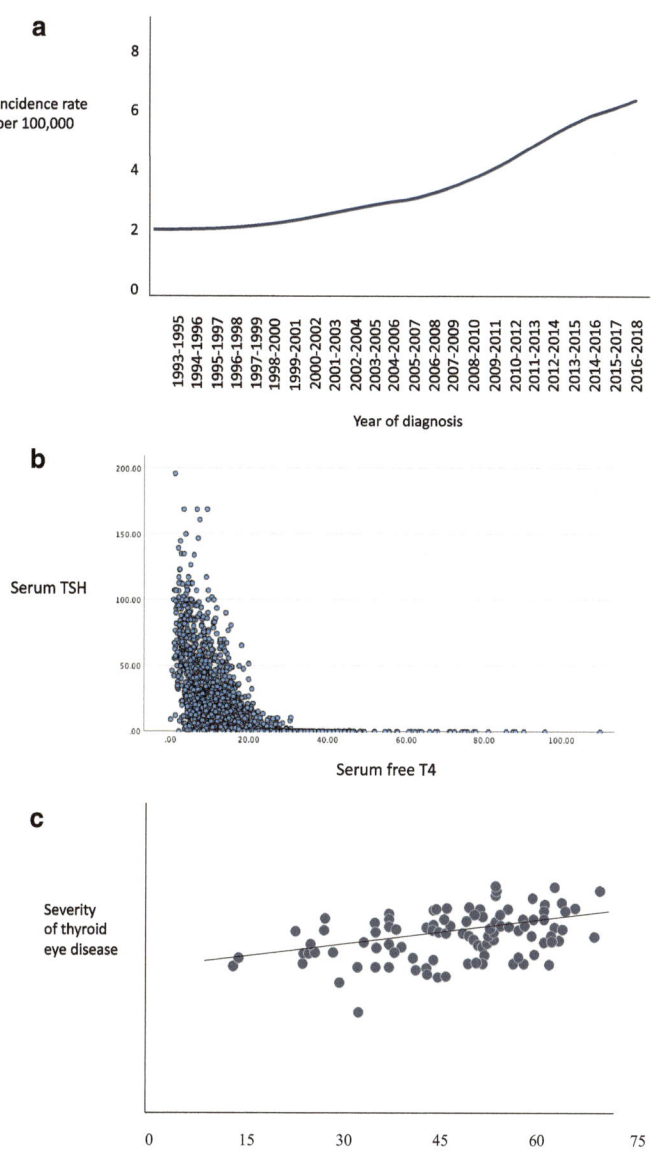

Fig. 6.8 (a) Correlation between annual incidence of thyroid cancers. (b) Negative correlation between levels of TSH and free T4. (c) Correlation between severity of thyroid eye disease and age of patients. (Attributions: A, B and C were redrawn from Cancer Research UK [20], Perros et al. [21], and Perros et al. [19])

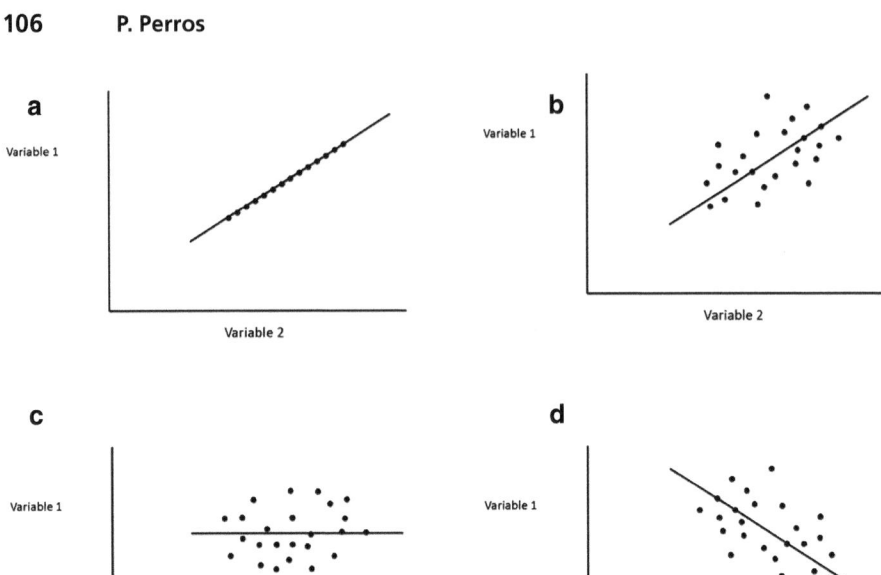

Fig. 6.9 Correlations between two sets of data. (**a**) Perfect correlation with a correlation coefficient (*r*) of 1. (**b**) *r* = 0.8 (respectable correlation). (**c**) *r* = 0 (no correlation). (**d**) *r* = -0.8 (respectable negative correlation)

Checklist

Interpretation Checklist
- The findings in the paper are 'clinically' important.
- The balance between efficacy and safety of a treatment is favourable.
- The cost of treatment is proportionate to the benefit.
- The data cannot be explained differently from what the authors suggest.
- The conclusions derived from the data can be extrapolated to the general population.
- The data do not ring 'too good to be true' alarm bells.

Notes for Interpretation Checklist

Are the Differences Presented 'Clinically' Important?

Intuition

'Clinically' important means, does it make a material difference to the person on the receiving end? Sometimes we just know whether something matters or not. Last time I flew with a budget airline, it took 7 h from leaving home to touching down at the destination airport. It made me ponder whether the extra cost for priority boarding was worth the fuss. It reduced the time from starting to queue for boarding to bum on seat by about half an hour, but the fact was that all passengers arrived, priority or not, at the destination at exactly the same time. For me (and I suspect the majority of passengers) priority boarding made no difference to the total travel time from home to landing.

Minimally Important Change

Consider another example. A fizzy drink was found to have 0.0001% more sugar than another. This difference was highly statistically significant, but can our taste buds tell the difference and does it matter for our long-term health? Just because we can measure something with great precision and identify tiny differences does not mean it is worth responding to it.

In recent years the concept of 'minimally important change' has been increasingly adopted among researchers. Like the fizzy drinks, it makes the point that a statistically significant difference is often not enough to guide us to make decisions. If a drug reduces the amount of protrusion of the eyes of patients with thyroid eye disease by 0.5 mm, does that matter to the patient? And what about if it is 2 or 4 mm? There are ways of defining what is the minimum amount of reduction in protrusion that makes a difference to the patient. Unfortunately the minimally important change is often not known (because the necessary research has not been done), and this information is usually missing from papers, but when it is available, it is a bonus.

Bringing Stats into the Scene: Effect Size

Statistical analyses can help answer the question of whether significant differences are important in real life by providing numerical information about the 'effect size'. For example, my colleague who measured the size of the thyroid gland in women during and after pregnancy found a difference, but it is equally important to know how big is the difference. One can just look at the average sizes of the thyroid gland during and after pregnancy and state that on average the thyroid gland during pregnancy is 1.5 times larger than after. Stats can do a lot better than that by taking into account not only the averages but also the spread of the data.

For continuous variables (like the volume of the thyroid gland), 'Cohen's d' scores can be calculated that provide an idea of the effect size (e.g. a d score of 0.2 is considered a small effect size, 0.5 medium and 0.8 large). This allows meaningful comparisons of the effect size between studies on the same topic. For categorical data, statistics can provide similarly useful estimates of the effect size by working out 'relative risk', 'odds ratio', 'number needed to treat' and 'area under the curve'.

So, statistics can provide insight into the important question of 'effect size'.

Surrogate Measures

I spent the summer of 1981 in Borneo doing my medical student elective. One weekend I went on a long trek through the jungle with friends and a couple of Dayak guides. During one of our stops for a rest, I asked one of the guides how long it would take to reach our destination. His answer was '*two cigarettes*'. That was the local currency for measuring time. It took into account that on average the party stopped for a rest (and a cigarette for the guides) every 3 h and that progress was roughly steady and at a more or less constant pace. That is 'surrogate'. A substitute for the real thing, but roughly equivalent.

What we measure and how it relates to what we regard as important really matters. Certain outcomes are important without much discussion. If you have cancer, failure of the treatment to eradicate the cancer, cancer recurrence after treatment and death are hard outcomes.

In medical research 'surrogate measures' are used frequently as convenient substitutes to harder outcomes relevant to the question of what is clinically important. Since we are on the topic of cancer, one such surrogate measure of cancer treatment in patients with advanced disease is 'progression-free survival'. Progression-free survival is time lapsed after treatment during which patients are being monitored and shown that the cancer has not grown larger.

Progression of cancer occurs much earlier than death; hence, recurrence-free survival is used widely as a surrogate measure of effectiveness of treatments. However, many cancer drugs that improve progression-free survival have subsequently turned out not to prolong overall survival [22].

Another example from the thyroid field is the use of combination treatment (levothyroxine plus liothyronine) for hypothyroidism. It has been shown that some patients on levothyroxine treatment have T3 levels at the low end of the normal range [23]. Raising the T3 levels in the bloodstream of patients with hypothyroidism to the upper end of the range has been argued to be an important treatment goal [24]. Yet, several studies have shown that doing so by using combination treatment has no impact on patients' quality of life, symptoms, memory, mood, cognitive function or general wellbeing [25–32]. On such evidence it would seem that a high normal T3 level is an unreliable surrogate measure of success of treatment.

The downsides of surrogate measures, like progression-free survival and T3 levels outlined above, are the reasons why we should care whether what is being measured really matters. It is also the reason why many studies today include 'patient-reported outcomes' such as the quality of life.

Risk and Proportionality

People who are scared of flying are usually presented with figures that will hopefully reassure them. For instance, the Civil Aviation Authority states that *'there is an average of one fatality for every 287 million passengers carried by UK operators. This can be compared with a one in 19 million chance of being struck and killed by lightning in the UK or a one in 17,000 chance of being killed in a road accident'* [33]. You can, of course, reduce that chance to 0 by not flying, but it makes no logical sense, especially as everyday life involves taking tiny risks that are greater than flying, like crossing the road.

One common topic of discussion for people who have been diagnosed with thyroid cancer is whether radioactive iodine ablation after thyroid surgery is safe, especially with regard to the risk of another cancer developing later. Data from a large study show that there is a statistically significant association between having radioactive iodine treatment and developing another cancer [34]. But the risk of another cancer is low at 12 patients out of 1000 treated over 9 years, compared to 8 out of 1000 who did not have radioactive iodine. The other side of the equation is that the risk of the thyroid cancer recurring (for those cancer patients who are selected as candidates for radioactive iodine treatment) is generally 1 in 10 over 10 years. Therefore, in proportion to 1 in 10 risk of recurrence (which is halved by radioactive iodine treatment), the small excess risk of another cancer (4 in 1000) is seen by most experts and patients as worth taking. Risk and proportionality are therefore important concepts that need to be kept in mind in addition to whether the stats show a significant difference or not.

Is the Balance Between Efficacy and Safety Favourable?

While the health benefits of treatments may range from neutral to highly effective, no treatment is without risks. Some treatments for cancer are very effective in eradicating cancer, but their side effects are too severe to justify their use. Studies that evaluate treatments should address the balance between how effective the treatment is (efficacy) against the side effects (safety). This is not an easy task and will always be subjective to some extent. Ratios, percentages and numbers needed to treat provide information about efficacy. There are accepted ways of classifying side effects of treatments that help evaluate safety and compare different treatments [35]. Interpreting the evidence includes judging whether the authors' opinions about the balance between efficacy and safety are appropriate and convincing.

Is the Cost of Treatment Proportionate to the Benefit?

Our resources allocated to healthcare are finite; thus, there is always a degree of rationing in healthcare delivery. The balance between how effective the treatment is and its cost is 'cost-effectiveness'. It is not unusual for cost-effectiveness not to be addressed by papers on treatments. Sometimes the treatment has not yet been licensed, and there is no price tag attached. Secondary publications (e.g. guidelines) do have to address this issue, which is becoming increasingly difficult as the pharmaceutical industry and investors in health technologies stride forward at an ever-increasing pace, and it seems that prices of new and effective drugs are fixed largely by market forces. Organisations like the National Institute of Health and Care Excellence have developed sophisticated methods for calculating cost-effectiveness and apply them for approval of new treatments for funding by the state.

In the thyroid field, one of the most spectacular newcomers is a new drug for thyroid eye disease called Teprotumumab. It is highly effective and relatively safe, but the cost in the USA (only country where it is currently licensed) is $350,000 per patient [36]. There are no data on cost-effectiveness of this drug as yet, but sales in the USA reached $4 billion in the first 2 years since licensing.

Is There More Than One Interpretation of the Data?

Consider your understanding of the data and that of the authors. Are there any additional possible interpretations that the authors have not taken into account? Could there have been other contributors that may have biased the result?

Can the Conclusions Derived from the Data Be Extrapolated to the General Population that They Are Supposed to Represent?

Consider a study of hypothyroid patients that shows that 50% are male and have an average age at which the diagnosis was made of 65 years. We know from numerous large studies that 90% of hypothyroid patients are women and that they are usually diagnosed in their 40s or 50s. In this example, the sample seems to be highly unusual, and any conclusions reached may only apply to older male hypothyroid patients, not the average patient with hypothyroidism.

Are the Claims 'Too Good to Be True'?

In medicine there are very few '100%' effective treatments, and there are certainly no '100%' safe treatments. In fact most are nowhere near the 100% mark. I think we generally appreciate that hyperbolic claims are suspect and advertisers have wisen up to it. Remember '8 out of 10 cat owners prefer…'? It is more believable than 10 out of 10 cat owners. One recent example from the thyroid field was a paper that claimed 93.1% effectiveness of a drug for thyroid eye disease with 0 serious side effects. It was later retracted [37].

Levels of Evidence

Systematic reviews and guidelines try to synthesise all the available evidence and assign an overall score that is meaningful and can aid in decision-making. There are several such schemes. One often used classifies evidence about interventions into three main categories and gives an idea of the quality characteristics of publications [38].

- Level I (at least one high-quality randomised controlled study)
- Level II
    - Level II.1 (at least one high-quality, non-randomised controlled study)
    - Level II.2 (a case-control study or cohort study)
    - Level II.3 (multiple time-series studies or important results from large uncontrolled studies)
- Level III (expert opinions)

Putting It All Together

You can use the same strategy as in Chap. 5 to rate your interpretation of the paper. You can place a tick or a cross depending on whether the criterion described is satisfied or not. Sum up all the ticks and work out the percentage ([ticks/ticks + crosses] × 100). You will end up with a figure between 0 and 100%. The closer to the top the of the scale, the more likely that the publication is of good quality and the reverse (Fig. 6.10).

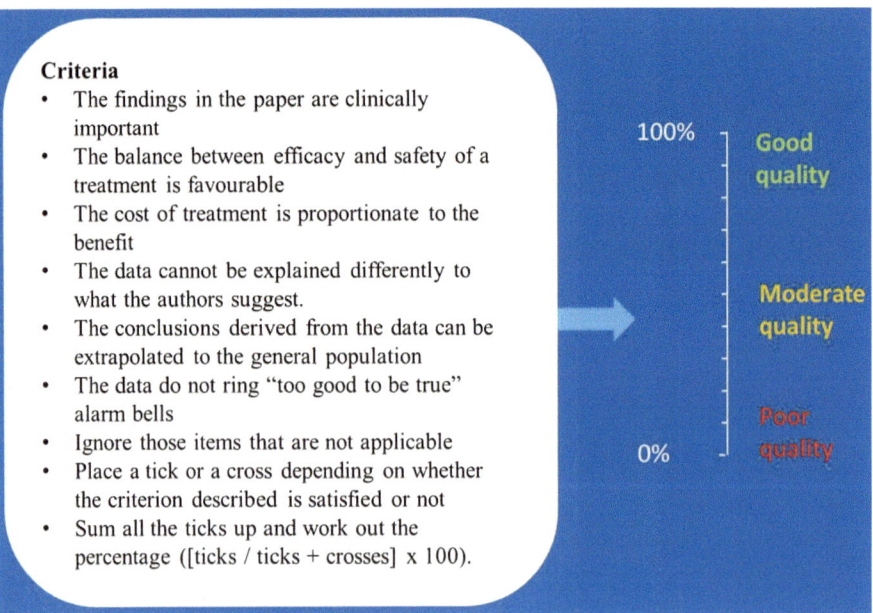

Criteria
- The findings in the paper are clinically important
- The balance between efficacy and safety of a treatment is favourable
- The cost of treatment is proportionate to the benefit
- The data cannot be explained differently to what the authors suggest.
- The conclusions derived from the data can be extrapolated to the general population
- The data do not ring "too good to be true" alarm bells
- Ignore those items that are not applicable
- Place a tick or a cross depending on whether the criterion described is satisfied or not
- Sum all the ticks up and work out the percentage ([ticks / ticks + crosses] x 100).

100%   Good quality

Moderate quality

0%   Poor quality

Fig. 6.10 Summary of interpretation checklist

End of the Journey

You have reached the end (Fig. 6.11). I hope you feel that you are now better equipped to find and wrestle with the evidence and get a little closer to the truth. You can test your new skills straight away by reading Part III where I pass verdict on four publications. See whether you agree.

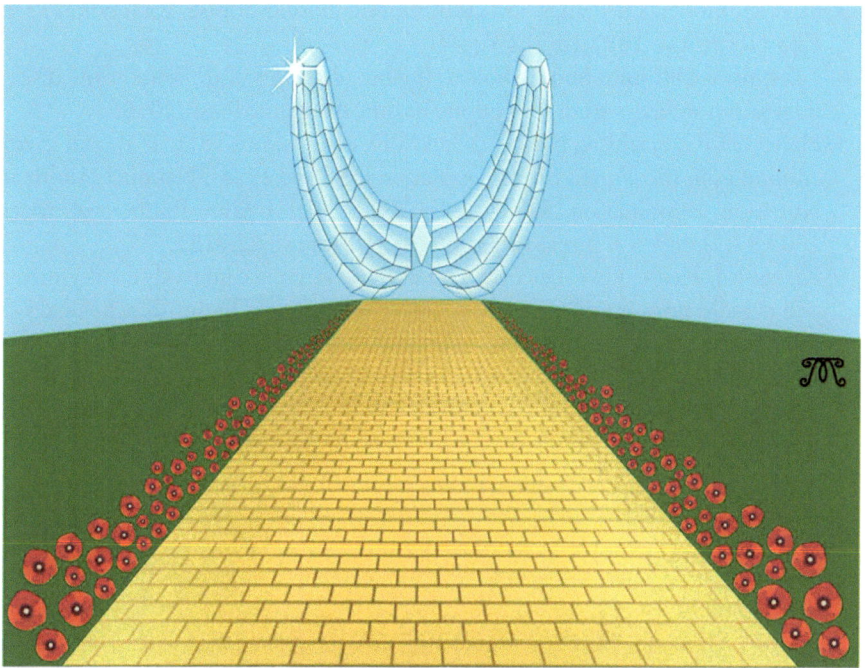

Fig. 6.11 Having a diagnosis plunges us into a torrent of uncertainty. Knowledge and understanding can help us move on the yellow brick road

References

1. Sun BJ, Li T, Mu Y, et al. Thyroid hormone modulates offspring sex ratio in a turtle with temperature-dependent sex determination. Proc Biol Sci. 2016;283(1841):20161206. https://doi.org/10.1098/rspb.2016.1206.
2. Perros P, Weightman DR, Crombie AL, Kendall-Taylor P. Azathioprine in the treatment of thyroid-associated ophthalmopathy. Acta Endocrinol (Copenh). 1990;122(1):8–12. https://doi.org/10.1530/acta.0.1220008.
3. Salvi M, How J. Pregnancy and autoimmune thyroid disease. Endocrinol Metab Clin North Am. 1987;16(2):431–44.
4. Tulchinsky TH. John Snow, cholera, the broad street pump; waterborne diseases then and now. Case studies in public health. Academic Press; 2018.
5. Hollowell JG, Staehling NW, Flanders WD, et al. Serum TSH, T(4), and thyroid antibodies in the United States population (1988 to 1994): National Health and Nutrition Examination Survey (NHANES III). J Clin Endocrinol Metab. 2002;87(2):489–99. https://doi.org/10.1210/jcem.87.2.8182.
6. Kratzsch J, Fiedler GM, Leichtle A, et al. New reference intervals for thyrotropin and thyroid hormones based on National Academy of Clinical Biochemistry criteria and regular ultrasonography of the thyroid. Clin Chem. 2005;51(8):1480–6. https://doi.org/10.1373/clinchem.2004.047399.
7. Jonklaas J, Razvi S. Reference intervals in the diagnosis of thyroid dysfunction: treating patients not numbers. Lancet Diabetes Endocrinol. 2019;7(6):473–83. https://doi.org/10.1016/S2213-8587(18)30371-1.
8. Andersen S, Pedersen KM, Bruun NH, Laurberg P. Narrow individual variations in serum T(4) and T(3) in normal subjects: a clue to the understanding of subclinical thyroid disease. J Clin Endocrinol Metab. 2002;87(3):1068–72. https://doi.org/10.1210/jcem.87.3.8165.
9. Perros P, Mason D, Pearce M, Pearce SHS, Chandler R, Mallick UK. Differentiated thyroid cancer mortality by disease stage in northern England. Clin Endocrinol (Oxf). 2020;93(1):61–6. https://doi.org/10.1111/cen.14187.
10. Roy A, Laszkowska M, Sundstrom J, et al. Prevalence of celiac disease in patients with autoimmune thyroid disease: a meta-analysis. Thyroid. 2016;26(7):880–90. https://doi.org/10.1089/thy.2016.0108.
11. Thvilum M, Brandt F, Almind D, Christensen K, Brix TH, Hegedus L. Increased psychiatric morbidity before and after the diagnosis of hypothyroidism: a nationwide register study. Thyroid. 2014;24(5):802–8. https://doi.org/10.1089/thy.2013.0555.
12. Taylor PN, Albrecht D, Scholz A, et al. Global epidemiology of hyperthyroidism and hypothyroidism. Nat Rev Endocrinol. 2018;14(5):301–16. https://doi.org/10.1038/nrendo.2018.18.
13. Zimmermann MB, Boelaert K. Iodine deficiency and thyroid disorders. Lancet Diabetes Endocrinol. 2015;3(4):286–95. https://doi.org/10.1016/S2213-8587(14)70225-6.

14. Hill AB. The environment and disease: association or causation? Proc R Soc Med. 1965;58(5):295–300.
15. Wiersinga WM. Smoking and thyroid. Clin Endocrinol (Oxf). 2013;79(2):145–51. https://doi.org/10.1111/cen.12222.
16. Pfeilschifter J, Ziegler R. Smoking and endocrine ophthalmopathy: impact of smoking severity and current vs lifetime cigarette consumption. Clin Endocrinol (Oxf). 1996;45(4):477–81. https://doi.org/10.1046/j.1365-2265.1996.8220832.x.
17. Davies L, Welch HG. Increasing incidence of thyroid cancer in the United States, 1973–2002. JAMA. 2006;295(18):2164–7. https://doi.org/10.1001/jama.295.18.2164.
18. Nagy EV, Perros P, Papini E, Katko M, Hegedus L. New formulations of levothyroxine in the treatment of hypothyroidism: trick or treat? Thyroid. 2021;31(2):193–201. https://doi.org/10.1089/thy.2020.0515.
19. Perros P, Crombie AL, Matthews JN, Kendall-Taylor P. Age and gender influence the severity of thyroid-associated ophthalmopathy: a study of 101 patients attending a combined thyroid-eye clinic. Clin Endocrinol (Oxf). 1993;38(4):367–72. https://doi.org/10.1111/j.1365-2265.1993.tb00516.x.
20. CancerResearch_Thyroid. https://www.cancerresearchuk.org/health-professional/cancer-statistics/statistics-by-cancer-type/thyroid-cancer/incidence#heading-Two.
21. Perros P, Basu A, Boelaert K, et al. Postradioiodine Graves' management: the PRAGMA study. Clin Endocrinol (Oxf). 2022;97(5):664–75. https://doi.org/10.1111/cen.14719.
22. Tannock IF, Pond GR, Booth CM. Biased evaluation in cancer drug trials—How use of progression-free survival as the primary end point can mislead. JAMA Oncol. 2022;8(5):679–80. https://doi.org/10.1001/jamaoncol.2021.8206.
23. Ito M, Miyauchi A, Hisakado M, et al. Biochemical markers reflecting thyroid function in athyreotic patients on levothyroxine monotherapy. Thyroid. 2017;27(4):484–90. https://doi.org/10.1089/thy.2016.0426.
24. Salvatore D, Porcelli T, Ettleson MD, Bianco AC. The relevance of T(3) in the management of hypothyroidism. Lancet Diabetes Endocrinol. 2022;10(5):366–72. https://doi.org/10.1016/S2213-8587(22)00004-3.
25. Appelhof BC, Fliers E, Wekking EM, et al. Combined therapy with levothyroxine and liothyronine in two ratios, compared with levothyroxine monotherapy in primary hypothyroidism: a double-blind, randomized, controlled clinical trial. J Clin Endocrinol Metab. 2005;90(5):2666–74. https://doi.org/10.1210/jc.2004-2111.
26. Clyde PW, Harari AE, Getka EJ, Shakir KM. Combined levothyroxine plus liothyronine compared with levothyroxine alone in primary hypothyroidism: a randomized controlled trial. JAMA. 2003;290(22):2952–8. https://doi.org/10.1001/jama.290.22.2952.

27. Escobar-Morreale HF, Botella-Carretero JI, Gomez-Bueno M, Galan JM, Barrios V, Sancho J. Thyroid hormone replacement therapy in primary hypothyroidism: a randomized trial comparing L-thyroxine plus liothyronine with L-thyroxine alone. Ann Intern Med. 2005;142(6):412–24. https://doi.org/10.7326/0003-4819-142-6-200503150-00007.

28. Rodriguez T, Lavis VR, Meininger JC, Kapadia AS, Stafford LF. Substitution of liothyronine at a 1:5 ratio for a portion of levothyroxine: effect on fatigue, symptoms of depression, and working memory versus treatment with levothyroxine alone. Endocr Pract. 2005;11(4):223–33. https://doi.org/10.4158/EP.11.4.223.

29. Saravanan P, Simmons DJ, Greenwood R, Peters TJ, Dayan CM. Partial substitution of thyroxine (T4) with tri-iodothyronine in patients on T4 replacement therapy: results of a large community-based randomized controlled trial. J Clin Endocrinol Metab. 2005;90(2):805–12. https://doi.org/10.1210/jc.2004-1672.

30. Sawka AM, Gerstein HC, Marriott MJ, MacQueen GM, Joffe RT. Does a combination regimen of thyroxine (T4) and 3,5,3'-triiodothyronine improve depressive symptoms better than T4 alone in patients with hypothyroidism? Results of a double-blind, randomized, controlled trial. J Clin Endocrinol Metab. 2003;88(10):4551–5. https://doi.org/10.1210/jc.2003-030139.

31. Siegmund W, Spieker K, Weike AI, et al. Replacement therapy with levothyroxine plus triiodothyronine (bioavailable molar ratio 14:1) is not superior to thyroxine alone to improve well-being and cognitive performance in hypothyroidism. Clin Endocrinol (Oxf). 2004;60(6):750–7. https://doi.org/10.1111/j.1365-2265.2004.02050.x.

32. Valizadeh M, Seyyed-Majidi MR, Hajibeigloo H, Momtazi S, Musavinasab N, Hayatbakhsh MR. Efficacy of combined levothyroxine and liothyronine as compared with levothyroxine monotherapy in primary hypothyroidism: a randomized controlled trial. Endocr Res. 2009;34(3):80–9. https://doi.org/10.1080/07435800903156340.

33. CAA. https://www.caa.co.uk/consumers/guide-to-aviation/aviation-safety/.

34. Brown AP, Chen J, Hitchcock YJ, Szabo A, Shrieve DC, Tward JD. The risk of second primary malignancies up to three decades after the treatment of differentiated thyroid cancer. J Clin Endocrinol Metab. 2008;93(2):504–15. https://doi.org/10.1210/jc.2007-1154.

35. CTCAE. https://ctep.cancer.gov/protocoldevelopment/electronic_applications/docs/CTCAE_v5_Quick_Reference_8.5x11.pdf.

36. Perros P, Hegedus L. Teprotumumab in thyroid eye disease: wonder drug or great divider? Eur Thyroid J. 2023;12(4):e230043. https://doi.org/10.1530/ETJ-23-0043.

37. Ye X, Zhao H, Liu J, Lu B, Shao J, Wang J. Retraction: efficacy and safety of tripterygium glycosides for active moderate to severe Graves' ophthalmopathy: a randomised, observer-masked, single-centre trial. Eur J Endocrinol. 2021;184(4):Z1. https://doi.org/10.1530/EJE-20-0857z.

38. USPreventiveServicesTaskForceProcedureManual. https://www.uspreventiveservicestaskforce.org/uspstf/sites/default/files/inline-files/procedure-manual_2016%20%281%29.pdf.

Part III

An Opinion

7

What Is the Optimal Range?

> 'Poor hypothyroidism control is the most serious and important area in the thyroid field that is in need of improvement'.

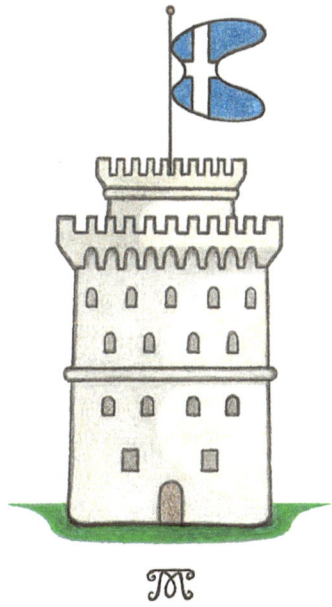

The White Tower is a landmark of Thessaloniki, the city I was born in. It owes its name to a convict who whitewashed the tower in exchange for his freedom in 1890. Before then it was known as the Red tower because of a massacre that took place in 1826. Earlier names included Tower of Kalamaria and Lions Tower, each name revealing some truth about its past. Like the White Tower the truth about the thyroid has many facets

The original version of the chapter has been revised. A correction to this chapter can be found at
https://doi.org/10.1007/978-3-031-58287-5_8

P. Perros, *Seeking Thyroid Truths*, Copernicus Books,
https://doi.org/10.1007/978-3-031-58287-5_7

Opinion Time

So far I have tried to refrain from sharing my own opinions about thyroid truths. I will not deny it, I may have faltered in some corner of preceding chapters and I am sure discerning readers will have picked that up. In this part of the book, my opinions will be expressed unapologetically. There are two reasons for this. Firstly, the topic of 'optimal range' is something close to my heart, and I have strong feelings about it. Secondly, it is a challenge and an opportunity for the reader to test what this book may have taught them and judge my opinions.

Part III focuses on the optimal range for serum TSH in hypothyroid patients who are taking levothyroxine medication. This is an area full of booby traps and controversies. Some patients on levothyroxine have persistent symptoms and may experiment with the dose of levothyroxine or add liothyronine tablets or desiccated thyroid extract. That is understandable and can explain why their serum TSH may be outside the reference range. The optimal range for such patients is a topic that deserves an entire separate book and is not covered by this chapter.

Here I want to focus on patients with hypothyroidism who are on levothyroxine treatment only and who do not consider themselves to have persistent symptoms that are connected to hypothyroidism. This makes up 85–90% of patients with a diagnosis of hypothyroidism.

Before I transform into my opinionated alter ego, I would like to introduce someone to you, who is the reason why Part III features in this book.

Laszlo, My Non-fiddle-Playing Nordic Friend

Laszlo, unlike me, is a proper academic, whose surname means fiddle-player in Hungarian, though, to the best of my knowledge, he is not a violinist. Like me, not only is he a sceptic, he enjoys being one. If the value of a piece of research is to be graded by its potential benefit on the health of the maximum number of people, then for me, Laszlo's work on the link between control of hypothyroidism and morbidity and mortality published in 2018 [1] is one that definitely meets this criterion.

Laszlo resisted my prompts for making more noise about this finding from him and his team when it was confirmed by an independent study in the UK a year later [2]. As I predicted, my suggestion was questioned with protestations, reminders of my previous misguided proposals, catastrophic events in human history and references to behaviours of primitive life forms. But admittedly on the few occasions when I succeeded in persuading him that my propositions have a solid basis, he has embraced them with uncharacteristic enthusiasm for a Dane or Swede or Hungarian (not sure which describes him best, as he was born in Hungary, lives in Denmark, but uses a Swedish passport). So my idea of publishing a commentary on this topic was critiqued, strip-searched, exposed and deconstructed by Laszlo's deliberations before an agreement was reached to go ahead. Annoyingly his prediction that journals would not find this message particularly 'sexy' and would resist publication was right. It took several attempts, and it has only been cited a handful of times since publication [3].

Laszlo's resistance to making a fuss about his research findings was not because of a hyperbolic sense of humility but because he had already tried by publishing and publicising his findings in the medical literature, by speaking in national and international meetings and by interacting with patients. The conclusions from his research about the optimal range had worked their way into international guidelines. Yet, the problem has not gone away, and the optimal range continues to evade many doctors and fails many patients. It was clear to Laszlo that another article in the medical press flagging up the same message would have been futile, and if the problem was to be fixed, other solutions had to be sought.

To put some context on the significance of achieving a normal serum TSH by hypothyroid patients on levothyroxine, it will help to think of the hypothyroidism-diabetes analogy.

The Hypothyroidism-Diabetes Analogy

There are many similarities between hypothyroidism and type 1 diabetes. Both have (for the most part) an autoimmune basis and lack important hormones, and their treatment involves hormonal replacement.

It was known for a long time that running a high or a low blood sugar level was associated with bad long-term outcomes including death, heart attacks, strokes, kidney failure, damage to nerve endings, blindness, cognitive impairment and all other rarer complications of diabetes. And for many years, doctors and patients with type 1 diabetes strived to keep the blood sugar within range, though it must be said generally with limited success. The uncertainty about whether such efforts were worthwhile was part of the problem. What was not clear was whether 'tight' control was overall beneficial ('tight' meaning getting the blood sugar as close to the normal range as possible). Bear in mind that the experience was that the tighter the control, the higher the risk of a low blood sugar (hypoglycaemia), which is another evil associated with complications, sometimes devastating. Another similarity between hypothyroidism and diabetes is that in both conditions there are reliable indirect measures of overall control. In hypothyroidism, the blood level of TSH, in diabetes 'glycated haemoglobin', was otherwise known as 'HbA1c'.

In 1993 a ground-breaking study was published in the *New England Journal of Medicine*, known as the Diabetes Control and Complications Trial (DCCT) [4]. It took an enormous amount of effort and resources to complete it. Nearly 1500 patients with type 1 diabetes were studied and treated with meticulous care. It involved 29 research centres, 6 years of recruitment (1983–1989) and another 4 years until follow-up was complete, and analyses were performed before it was finally published. For the first time, there was robust and conclusive evidence that intensive treatment that kept the HbA1c close to normal prevented diabetic complications. The results were announced with the customary US-style razmataz, flamboyance and drumrolls, and it remains one of the landmark studies of the late twentieth century. Deservedly so, the DCCT has been cited more than 17,000 times in the medical literature. The subsequent changes in medical practice have saved many lives and spared misery for millions of people with diabetes.

In the thyroid field, we always lag behind diabetes and we don't quite manage to mirror the advances in diabetes research. I think the main reasons are that hypothyroidism is not seen as serious a condition as diabetes (and to be fair that is true), and the complications of poor thyroid control are not as frequent or severe as in diabetes. For these and no doubt other reasons, I expect that there will never be an HCCT (Hypothyroidism Control and Complications Trial). But there is already a compelling body of evidence about outcomes of poorly controlled hypothyroidism that cannot be ignored. Yet it has attracted little attention, while misinformation belittling the potentially harmful effects of overtreatment (as mirrored by a low serum level of TSH) bounces liberally around the echo chambers of some patient blogs [5–7]. This is a matter that makes me agitated and animated, and I have saved it to the end of this book hoping to attract more of the reader's attention.

Many People with Hypothyroidism Have Poor Control

Several cross-sectional studies have shown a high frequency of serum TSH values falling outside the normal reference range (27–41% low TSH 11.2–16% high TSH) and in total 37.2–57% of patients with hypothyroidism being treated with levothyroxine have an abnormal level of TSH at any one time [8–10]. A study from the Netherlands has shown that even those patients who hit the target with a normal serum TSH, have a 19–24% chance of drifting outside the normal range, if their TSH is re-tested 6 weeks later [11]. In the context of the Dutch findings, it makes one wonder how appropriate is the standard practice by most family doctors of checking thyroid blood tests of hypothyroid patients once every 1 or 2 years.

Implications of Abnormal Serum TSH in Levothyroxine-Treated People with Hypothyroidism

In Chap. 5, reproducibility of studies and 'Rawlin's law' was mentioned whereby a minimum of two independent studies pointing in the same direction is required for findings to be considered credible. So, a single study suggests that a result is plausible, two concurring studies makes it likely, three almost certain and four are a rare luxury. On the topic of associations between abnormal serum TSH with outcomes, not one, not two, not three, but four large-scale studies have been published with concordant results [1, 2, 8, 12].

The message is the same, though some variation in detail is inevitably present. If you are taking levothyroxine and you are running a serum TSH outside the normal range, you are at risk of premature death and cardiovascular complications. A rough calculation based on the prevalence of hypothyroidism in the general population (about 5%), and assuming that approximately half of levothyroxine-treated patients at any one time have an abnormal TSH leads to the conclusion that about 18 million people in Europe are at risk of premature death and other complications because of this association. If we extrapolate this to the global population, those at risk reach 200 million. As the final touches to this book were being tidied up, a further bit of bad news was published. A low serum TSH in people over the age of 65 years being treated with thyroid hormones was associated with an excess risk of cognitive disorder [13].

You may recall from Chap. 1 the 'rooster syndrome'. Association is not necessarily causation; therefore, one has to exercise a degree of scepticism as to whether achieving a normal TSH can reverse the risks mentioned above. For this we need a large prospective randomised double-blind study, a 'Hypothyroidism Control and Complications Trial'. This I fear will never happen for the reasons outlined above, though I hope to be proven wrong. So we will have to content ourselves with what we have.

There are two important points relating to the associations between abnormal serum TSH and adverse outcomes: (a) there is what seems to be a 'dose-response' effect; in other words, the more one deviates from the normal TSH range and the longer the exposure, the higher the risk, which strengthens the probability of a causal relationship; (b) the size of the effect of an abnormal serum TSH on mortality seems to be small, but this is not necessarily reassuring as the number of people affected is huge.

Collateral Evidence

Are there any parallel examples on the impact of the level of control of hypothyroidism, as measured by the serum TSH that we can draw further insight from? There are indeed from the obstetric and paediatric worlds. These two phases of life (in the womb and in childhood) are particularly important because that is when intellectual and physical development take place most rapidly. Growth and development are processes that require an optimal hormonal environment and small disturbances, which may be inconsequential in adult life, can leave a permanent mark.

The experience from pregnancy is that maintenance of normal TSH in hypothyroid mothers on levothyroxine results in similar outcomes to the normal population, while deviations of serum TSH outside the range lead to adverse results [14]. The paediatric experience is similar. Children with congenital hypothyroidism who are treated with levothyroxine and achieve normal TSH do well and those who do not, fare worse [15–17].

The Rose Paradox

Geoffrey Rose was an English epidemiologist who designed the Whitehall study, which established links between mortality and a range of risk factors. One of Rose's contributions to epidemiology and public health was the 'Rose paradox', which states that 'a large number of people at small risk may give rise to more cases than a small number of people at high risk' [18]. Therefore, the small effect size of the potential consequences of poor control of hypothyroidism should not instil complacency, because Rose's paradox probably applies.

Normal and Optimal Range

The normal range for a blood test is usually defined statistically by the values of the healthy population. The limits are set at 95% of the results closest to the average. This definition of the normal range has been criticised for being meaningless and arbitrary. Another way of looking at what is an optimal range is to correlate it with health outcomes. The evidence already discussed indicates that at least for people with hypothyroidism who are being treated with levothyroxine, the optimal range seems to follow closely the normal TSH range. There is an argument that we should not be exclusively preoccupied by the TSH level and that it is more relevant to correlate blood levels of T3 and health outcomes. Unfortunately such studies are not available, and we probably will not know for a while whether some other parameters that reflect the thyroid status may predict outcomes better than the TSH level. That is no reason however to bury our heads in the sand and pretend that an abnormal TSH level does not matter.

What Needs to Be Done?

The reasons why the serum TSH drifts outside the normal range are multiple and complex. Often it has to do with how the levothyroxine tablets are taken. Food and drink (other than plain water) can interfere with the absorption of levothyroxine. Some medications if taken together with levothyroxine also impair absorption. Other medical conditions, such as atrophic gastritis, coeliac disease and other gut conditions, can interfere with absorption. Changing the brand of levothyroxine can also make a difference. Sometimes the healthcare professional gives wrong advice, or there is miscommunication. In a recent study, forgetfulness was the commonest cause and accounted for 22% of 'non-adherence' [19]. At this point, you might anticipate the doctor's finger of blame to point at the patient. The last time this doctor was prescribed medication it was antibiotics following a hand injury. He took the first dose of the day most days. He forgot the second dose most days, and as for the third dose, well you can guess. He stopped the course prematurely, because he was not convinced he needed them. The hand did not look infected, and there was no obvious benefit after 3 days of taking the pills. And by the way what did the GP know, she looked like she had just graduated from nursery. Besides, those intestinal grumbles after the second day were surely side effects.

It is possible to reduce non-adherence by using 'mediboxes', setting up reminders on smartphones and other similar strategies, but these interventions only work for some. If the expectation is for patients to follow advice about taking medication, they have to be much better informed than what is generally achieved in real practice. There needs to be trust, and the decision to start the medication must be taken jointly between the patient and doctor. And let us not forget other barriers, such as the fact that taking the medication serves as a reminder that a person has a chronic illness and is different from 'normal' people. New technologies and innovations about alternative ways of delivering thyroid hormones to the traditional tablet formulations may prove helpful. Diabetes provides another useful example. When self-measurement of blood glucose became available, control of diabetes improved for many. It illustrates how important it is for us to constantly have a feel of what we achieve when we try hard. Measurements of thyroid hormones using hand-held meters have already been developed and may have a role in reaching and maintaining good control. Most importantly, tackling the problem of poor hypothyroidism control needs to be approached by health professionals outside a 'blame' framework. There are always reasons why we don't take medications, and ineptitude or obstinance are rarely among them. While progress can be made for every individual patient by working together with health professionals, there is a wider need to raise awareness of the magnitude of poor control of hypothyroidism and its consequences as a public health problem.

It is my strong impression that poor hypothyroidism control, as defined by an abnormal TSH level, is the most serious and important area in the thyroid field that is in need of improvement. I am hopeful that patients, endocrinologists and their respective organisations will work together to attract and secure the resources needed in order to improve health outcomes for people with hypothyroidism.

References

1. Lillevang-Johansen M, Abrahamsen B, Jorgensen HL, Brix TH, Hegedus L. Over- and under-treatment of hypothyroidism is associated with excess mortality: a register-based cohort study. Thyroid. 2018;28(5):566–74. https://doi.org/10.1089/thy.2017.0517.
2. Thayakaran R, Adderley NJ, Sainsbury C, et al. Thyroid replacement therapy, thyroid stimulating hormone concentrations, and long term health outcomes in

patients with hypothyroidism: longitudinal study. BMJ. 2019;366:l4892. https://doi.org/10.1136/bmj.l4892.

3. Perros P, Nirantharakumar K, Hegedus L. Recent evidence sets therapeutic targets for levothyroxine-treated patients with primary hypothyroidism based on risk of death. Eur J Endocrinol. 2021;184(2):C1–3. https://doi.org/10.1530/EJE-20-1229.

4. Nathan DM, Genuth S, Lachin J, et al. The effect of intensive treatment of diabetes on the development and progression of long-term complications in insulin-dependent diabetes mellitus. N Engl J Med. 1993;329(14):977–86. https://doi.org/10.1056/NEJM199309303291401.

5. StopTheThyroidMadness. https://stopthethyroidmadness.com/tsh-why-its-useless/.

6. TPAUK. https://www.tpauk.com/main/article/on-the-clinical-diagnosis-and-treatment-of-hypothyroidism-2/.

7. ThyroidPatientAdvocacyUK. https://www.tpauk.com/main/article/on-the-clinical-diagnosis-and-treatment-of-hypothyroidism-2/.

8. Flynn RW, Bonellie SR, Jung RT, MacDonald TM, Morris AD, Leese GP. Serum thyroid-stimulating hormone concentration and morbidity from cardiovascular disease and fractures in patients on long-term thyroxine therapy. J Clin Endocrinol Metab. 2010;95(1):186–93. https://doi.org/10.1210/jc.2009-1625.

9. Somwaru LL, Arnold AM, Joshi N, Fried LP, Cappola AR. High frequency of and factors associated with thyroid hormone over-replacement and under-replacement in men and women aged 65 and over. J Clin Endocrinol Metab. 2009;94(4):1342–5. https://doi.org/10.1210/jc.2008-1696.

10. Okosieme OE, Belludi G, Spittle K, Kadiyala R, Richards J. Adequacy of thyroid hormone replacement in a general population. QJM. 2011;104(5):395–401. https://doi.org/10.1093/qjmed/hcq222.

11. Flinterman LE, Kuiper JG, Korevaar JC, et al. Impact of a forced dose-equivalent levothyroxine brand switch on plasma thyrotropin: a cohort study. Thyroid. 2020;30(6):821–8. https://doi.org/10.1089/thy.2019.0414.

12. Evron JM, Hummel SL, Reyes-Gastelum D, Haymart MR, Banerjee M, Papaleontiou M. Association of thyroid hormone treatment intensity with cardiovascular mortality among US veterans. JAMA Netw Open. 2022;5(5):e2211863. https://doi.org/10.1001/jamanetworkopen.2022.11863.

13. Adams R, Oh ES, Yasar S, Lyketsos CG, Mammen JS. Endogenous and exogenous thyrotoxicosis and risk of incident cognitive disorders in older adults. JAMA Intern Med. 2023;183:1324. Epub ahead of print. PMID: 37870843; PMCID: PMC10594176. https://doi.org/10.1001/jamainternmed.2023.5619.

14. Sullivan SA. Hypothyroidism in pregnancy. Clin Obstet Gynecol. 2019;62(2):308–19. https://doi.org/10.1097/GRF.0000000000000432.

15. van Trotsenburg P, Stoupa A, Leger J, et al. Congenital hypothyroidism: a 2020-2021 consensus guidelines update—an ENDO-European reference network initiative endorsed by the European Society for Pediatric Endocrinology

and the European Society for Endocrinology. Thyroid. 2021;31(3):387–419. https://doi.org/10.1089/thy.2020.0333.

16. Uyttendaele M, Lambert S, Tenoutasse S, et al. Congenital hypothyroidism: long-term experience with early and high levothyroxine dosage. Horm Res Paediatr. 2016;85(3):188–97. https://doi.org/10.1159/000443958.

17. Aleksander PE, Bruckner-Spieler M, Stoehr AM, et al. Mean high-dose L-thyroxine treatment is efficient and safe to achieve a normal IQ in young adult patients with congenital hypothyroidism. J Clin Endocrinol Metab. 2018;103(4):1459–69. https://doi.org/10.1210/jc.2017-01937.

18. Davies P, Jenkinson S. Interpreting the evidence. Student BMJ. 2008;16. https://doi.org/10.1136/sbmj.0801026.

19. Mehuys E, Lapauw B, T'Sjoen G, et al. Investigating levothyroxine use and its association with thyroid health in patients with hypothyroidism: a community pharmacy study. Thyroid. 2023;33(8):918–26. https://doi.org/10.1089/thy.2023.0066.

Correction to: What Is the Optimal Range?

Correction to:
Chapter 7 in: P. Perros, *Seeking Thyroid Truths*,
Copernicus Books,
https://doi.org/10.1007/978-3-031-58287-5_7

The figure in chapter opening page was incorrect. It has been updated in this corrected version.

The updated version of this chapter can be found at
https://doi.org/10.1007/978-3-031-58287-5_7

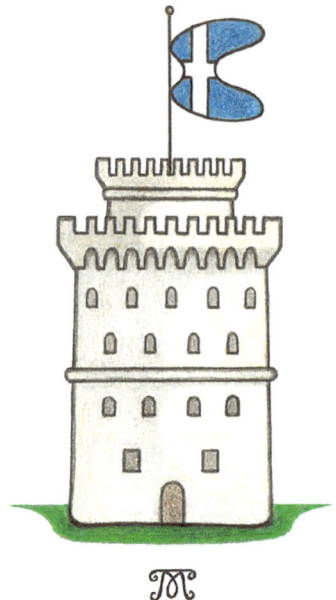

The White Tower is a landmark of Thessaloniki, the city I was born in. It owes its name to a convict who whitewashed the tower in exchange for his freedom in 1890. Before then it was known as the Red tower because of a massacre that took place in 1826. Earlier names included Tower of Kalamaria and Lions Tower, each name revealing some truth about its past. Like the White Tower the truth about the thyroid has many facets

Epilogue

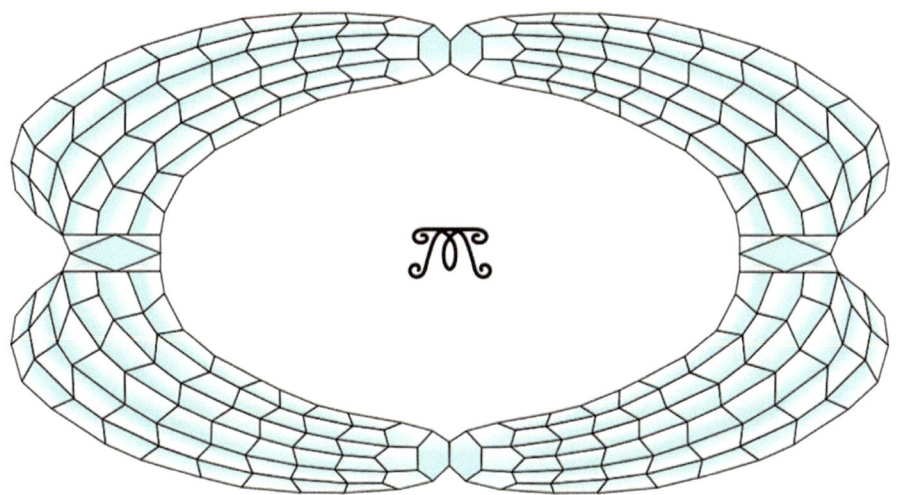

P. Perros, *Seeking Thyroid Truths*, Copernicus Books, https://doi.org/10.1007/978-3-031-58287-5

I started writing this book a couple of years before the COVID pandemic. It then fell by the wayside as other priorities and distractions prevailed. A few months before lockdown, my wife and I met Pat Kendall-Taylor, a friend who has also been a supervisor, colleague and mentor. My retirement was looming and Pat asked what my plans were. I confided in her that I had decided to write a book. We met again in the summer of 2022 at the Duke of Wellington in Newton near Hexham and she asked me how the book was coming along. My embarrassment proved to be the kick up the backside that was needed to lift me out of procrastination and postponement tactics, so I owe Pat a big thanks.

Finding the evidence and understanding what it means is only a small part of something much bigger. Generating the data upon which the evidence is based requires the labour of many experts from conception of an idea to performing the experiments and studies, processing the results and finally sharing them. We, as readers, are beneficiaries of this process and we learn and broaden our horizons. The irony is that when the evidence provides a solution to a serious health problem, implementation turns out to be the biggest hurdle.

Thyrish-English Lexicon

Abstract A brief summary of a *paper*.

Anatomy The structure and shape of a part of the body.

Antibody A protein made by the body's immune system that binds specifically (like lock and key) to another *protein* (*antigen*). Antibodies are made by the body when it is invaded by infections. Antibodies seek the bugs out and neutralise them. Most vaccines work by encouraging our body to make antibodies before they are infected. Antibodies are also used to measure *hormones* in the bloodstream. In *autoimmune thyroid* diseases, antibodies are made that attack the *thyroid* and can cause its destruction or make it overactive or underactive.

Antigen A chemical in the body (usually a *protein*) against which *antibodies* are made.

Anti-microsomal antibody Antibodies found in *autoimmune thyroid* disease. They are called 'microsomal' because they were initially detected by their ability to stick to 'microsomes', tiny structures inside cells. It is now known that these *antibodies* stick specifically to an *enzyme protein* called *thyroid peroxidase*, which is abundant in many cells including the *thyroid*. The microsomal antibody test has now been largely replaced by the *thyroid peroxidase antibody* test, as the latter is more reliable. A positive microsomal antibody or *thyroid peroxidase antibody test* indicates that there is an underlying *autoimmune* process against the *thyroid gland*.

Antioxidants Chemicals that neutralise *oxygen radicals*.

Assay A word that means a measurement. It refers to the method or the process of measuring a chemical, in some biological fluid, usually blood.

Association A statistical term which indicates that knowing about one parameter also tells us about another.

Atrial fibrillation A type of rapid irregular heart beat sometimes caused by *thyroid* overactivity.

P. Perros, *Seeking Thyroid Truths*, Copernicus Books,
https://doi.org/10.1007/978-3-031-58287-5

Autoantigen A chemical, usually a *protein* that is made in our body, but is targeted by our immune system.

Autoimmune Autoimmune conditions are a group of diseases whereby the body's defence system (immune system) against infections, turns against itself, fooled into thinking that the organ it attacks does not belong to the body.

Autoimmune hypothyroidism Also known as *Hashimoto's disease* or *Hashimoto's thyroiditis* refers to *hypothyroidism* due to *autoimmunity*. It is often accompanied by enlargement of the *thyroid gland* because of an accumulation of white cells within it and with positive *thyroid antibodies*.

Azathioprine A drug used in several *autoimmune* diseases, which suppresses the immune attack on tissues. Azathioprine has been used for *thyroid eye disease* in the past, but the evidence is unconvincing and other drug treatments for *thyroid eye disease* are now used in preference to azathioprine.

Basic research Laboratory-based experimental research.

Benign Non-cancerous.

Biopsy A sample of tissue taken from a patient, usually in order to help make a diagnosis.

Calcitonin A *hormone* produced by a separate type of cell to those producing *T3* and *T4* within the *thyroid gland*. The function of calcitonin is related to bone metabolism, especially during growth and development. In large doses, it has been used as a treatment for osteoporosis. It probably has no major role in adults.

Case-control study A type of study that looks at whether a group defined by a diagnosis or exposure to treatment or a risk factor, has an outcome that is different to a comparative control group; however, the control group has not entered the study at the same time or with the same criteria as the cases (subjects) that are being studied.

Case report A type of study describing something related to a single patient that is unusual and insightful.

Case series A type of study similar to a *case report* but contains a larger numbers of patients, usually from the same centre.

Categorical data Data that are sorted in groups, like male or female, alive or dead, child or adult.

Cervical Pertaining to the neck (cervix).

Citation The description of a published piece of academic work and usually includes the names of the authors, the title of the work, the name of the journal (or book, or website), year, issue number and page number.

Clinical Activity Score A method for judging how much inflammation there is in the back of the eyes of patients with *thyroid eye disease*.

Cohort study A type of study that focuses on populations with some common characteristic (e.g. patients with a diagnosis of *hypothyroidism*) and record data at baseline and at some subsequent interval(s).

Commentary A type of publication usually commissioned by the journal to an expert who puts forward his/her opinion on a *paper* that is published in the same issue of the journal.

Confidence interval A statistical term that describes the spread of values within which we expect the average to be.

Congenital hypothyroidism *Hypothyroidism* that is present from birth.

Compensated hypothyroidism Also called *subclinical hypothyroidism* is a subtle type of *thyroid* underactivity, which is so mild that it causes no symptoms and the diagnosis is made by blood tests. It is defined as a serum *TSH* above the upper limit of normal but less than 10 mU/litre, associated with a normal *FT4* level.

Consensus statement A type of publication similar to a *guideline*, but tends to cover areas in medicine where the evidence is scarce and therefore recommendations are based more on experience and expert opinion than robust evidence.

Continuous data Data that are measured on a continuous scale, such as age, size, price.

Control group A group of subjects participating in a study that are used for comparison to the 'test group' of participants.

Correlation A statistical term which indicates that a relationship between variables so that when one changes the other also alters proportionately.

Correlation coefficient A number that derives from a statistical analysis, which tells us how close the points are between the variables we are interested in, to a straight line.

Cost effectiveness The balance between how effective the treatment is and its cost.

Cretin/cretinism A condition that results from severe iodine deficiency and *hypothyroidism* in early life leading to intellectual impairment, stunted growth, hearing and speech defects, walking difficulties and some may have a goitre.

Cross-sectional study A study that collects information at one particular time (like a snapshot).

CRP Stands for C-reactive protein. It is a blood test that can tell doctors whether there is inflammation somewhere in the body. The CRP can be raised in *subacute thyroiditis*.

Cricoid cartilage A ring-shaped structure made of cartilage that sits above the *thyroid gland* in the neck.

Cyanobacteria A primitive form of bacteria that can use light for energy.

De Quervain thyroiditis Inflammation of the *thyroid* due to a viral infection. It is also called *subacute thyroiditis* or *viral thyroiditis*.

Derbyshire neck *Endemic goitre* in people who used to live in Derbyshire (now eradicated).

Double-blinded A type of study whereby neither patient nor researcher knows which treatment corresponds to which patient until the study is complete.

Editorial A publication in a journal written by one of the editors about some other publication, which usually represents the journal opinion.

Effect size The difference that an intervention (e.g. treatment) makes.

Efficacy Effectiveness of a drug or treatment.

Empirical knowledge Knowledge gathered by observation, experimentation, collection of facts and analysis.

Endemic A condition or disease that clusters in a confined geographical area.

Endocrine gland A *gland,* producing chemicals (*hormones*) that are released into the bloodstream, rather than to a particular part of the body outside the circulation.

Endocrinologist A specialist in *hormonal* diseases.

Enzyme Enzymes are proteins that act as 'catalysts'; in other words, they facilitate chemical reactions in the body. For instance, the breaking down of nutrients in food that can then be absorbed is carried out by enzymes. Meat tenderiser is an enzyme and fermentation that makes alcohol from sugar also requires enzymes that are found in yeasts.

ER Emergency room.

ESR Stands for erythrocyte sedimentation rate. It is a blood test that can tell doctors whether there is inflammation somewhere in the body. The ESR can be raised in *subacute thyroiditis.*

Exocrine gland A gland that releases its secretions to parts of the body other than the bloodstream (e.g. saliva, digestive juices, tears).

FT3 and FT4 The letter 'F' stands for 'free'. Most of the *T3* and *T4* that circulates in the bloodstream is packaged up with other *proteins,* thus leaving only a small fraction 'free' to pass from blood vessels to tissues. The bound *T3* and *T4* in the circulation acts as a reservoir of ready-made *hormones* that can be used immediately if needed. Modern *thyroid* blood tests measure the free fraction, which is the most representative.

Gland An organ that produces secretions.

Goitre An enlargement of the *thyroid gland,* thought to be derived from the Latin 'guttur', which means throat.

Graves' disease Named after the nineteenth century Irish physician Robert Graves who described it. It is an *autoimmune* disease whereby the body makes *antibodies* against the *TSH receptor* and drives the *thyroid* to produce excess amounts of *thyroid hormones* and cause *hyperthyroidism.*

Guideline A type of publication that uses all the available evidence, including *systematic reviews* and *meta-analyses,* to formulate recommendations on how patients should be managed in real life.

H-index Stands for 'Hirsch index' and is a metric for individual academics. It is calculated on the basis of how many times that person's *papers* have been cited by peers.

Hashimoto Hakaru Hashimoto was a Japanese scientist and doctor. He described 'struma lymphomatosa' in 1912 now commonly referred to as *Hashimoto's thyroiditis* or *Hashimoto's disease.*

Hashimoto's disease Also known as *Hashimoto's thyroiditis* or *autoimmune hypothyroidism* refers to *hypothyroidism* due to *autoimmunity.* It is often accompanied by enlargement of the *thyroid gland* because of an accumulation of white cells within it and with positive *thyroid antibodies*. Many otherwise healthy people may have Hashimoto's disease without any symptoms and with normally functioning *thyroid* glands, but are more at risk of developing an underactive *thyroid* in future. There is some evidence that *Hashimoto's disease* with the passage of time leads to shrinkage of the *thyroid gland* as it eventually becomes destroyed by the *autoimmune* process, which is referred to as *Ord's thyroiditis*.

Hashimoto's encephalopathy A diagnosis that is not universally accepted. 'Encephalopathy' is a generic term for malfunction of the brain and has numerous causes from infections to various organ failures, disturbances of blood levels of various chemicals, *autoimmunity*, drugs, the list is endless. Sometimes no cause can be found. *Hashimoto's encephalopathy* is used to describe cases of encephalopathy without a known cause when patients happen to have positive *thyroid antibodies*. Given that up to 15% of the population carries *thyroid antibodies*, the association with encephalopathy may be expected in about 15% of cases of encephalopathy of unknown cause.

Hashimoto's thyroiditis Also known as *Hashimoto's disease* or *autoimmune hypothyroidism* refers to *hypothyroidism* due to *autoimmunity* . It is often accompanied by enlargement of the *thyroid gland* because of an accumulation of white cells within it and with positive *thyroid antibodies*. Many otherwise healthy people may have Hashimoto's thyroiditis without any symptoms and with normally functioning thyroid glands, but are more at risk of developing an underactive *thyroid* in future. There is some evidence that Hashimoto's thyroiditis with the passage of time leads to shrinkage of the thyroid gland as it eventually becomes destroyed by the *autoimmune* process, which is referred to as *Ord's thyroiditis*.

Hashitoxicosis A relatively rare variant of *autoimmune thyroid* disease where *hypothyroidism* turns into *hyperthyroidism*. Such swings can continue to occur over several years.

Hormone A chemical messenger produced by *endocrine glands* in the body. *Hormones* are secreted into the bloodstream and reach other parts of the body where they have their effect. *T3, T4* and *calcitonin* are all *thyroid* hormones.

Hyperthyroid Overactive *thyroid*, a condition that has many causes, which leads to high levels of *thyroid hormones* in the bloodstream due to increased production of *thyroid hormones*.

Hypothesis An assumption or theory.

Hypothyroid *Underactive thyroid*, a condition that has many causes, which leads to low levels of *thyroid hormones* in the bloodstream.

Hypothalamus A small area of the brain above the *pituitary gland*, which controls many *endocrine glands* including the pituitary secretion of *TSH*.

Impact factor A quality metric for a journal, derived from the number of times publications in that journal are cited by other publications.

Interventional study A study of a treatment, procedure or device (the intervention).

Isthmus From the Greek ισθμος meaning a narrow strip of land connecting two larger pieces of land. In human anatomy, it is the narrow piece of *thyroid gland* that connects the two *thyroid* halves (*lobes*).

Letter to the editor A type of publication written by any reader of a journal who wishes to share a view, usually about a *paper* in the journal.

Liothyronine The name of the manufactured *thyroid hormone T3*. Liothyronine is chemically identical to *tri-iodothyronine*, the naturally occurring *thyroid hormone*.

Lipid membrane The outer wall of cells, as well as the lining of other important structures within cells.

Lobe A round or egg-like part of an organ. The *thyroid* has a right and a left lobe connected by the *isthmus*.

Lobotomy Brain surgery for mental illness.

Longitudinal study A study that follows patients up for a length of time.

Lymphocytes A type of white immune cells that in *autoimmune* diseases can damage tissues and cells.

Malignant Cancerous.

Mean, median, mode Statistical terms that describe the average in a set of data.

Meta-analysis A type of publication that uses valid statistical methods to combine the results from several similar studies.

Metabolism The chemical processed involved to maintain life.

Metamorphosis In biology, metamorphosis refers to the process of transformation that happens in some animals from a larva form to a mature adult. In amphibians, like the frog, metamorphosis refers to tadpoles turning into adult frogs. This process is regulated by *thyroid hormones*.

Minimal important change The minimum change in a measure that patients perceive as important.

Mutation A change in a gene that may cause a disease.

Myxoedema Another word for *hypothyroid*, but usually reserved for severe cases. 'Myxoedema' literally means swelling of tissue due to deposition of a mucous material.

Narrative review A type of publication that tells a story about a subject and original research that the authors consider relevant, upon which their interpretations and opinions are based.

Nodule A lump or swelling.

Null hypothesis The assumption that there is no significant difference between two groups of observations.

Observational study A study reporting on something interesting or unusual that happens.

Octreotide A drug that reduces the levels of growth hormone in the body. It was developed as a treatment for acromegaly (a rare condition due to a benign tumour of the *pituitary gland*). It was initially reported to be an effective treatment for *thyroid eye disease*, but subsequent studies showed that the effect was minimal or absent.

Ord's thyroiditis Named after William Ord, a nineteenth century physician who reported that the *thyroid glands* of patients with *myxoedema* were shrunken, scarred and infiltrated by white cells. This eponym is rarely used today.

Organotherapy A nineteenth century vogue for administering mushed up organs into patients as treatments for a variety of diseases.

Overt hypothyroidism Low blood levels of *T4*, associated with elevated *TSH* and usually accompanied by symptoms of *hypothyroidism*, to distinguish it from *subclinical hypothyroidism*.

Oxygen radicals Chemicals containing oxygen that are generated during production of *thyroid hormones*. They are highly reactive and can cause damage to cells unless neutralised by *thyroid peroxidase*.

Paper A scientific publication, or article in a journal.

Peer review The process whereby independent experts in the field scrutinise and approve scientific writings before they are published.

Peroxidase An *enzyme* that breaks up peroxide. *Thyroid* peroxidase is an enzyme found in the *thyroid gland* that is involved in making *thyroid hormones*. It is also an 'autoantigen'.

Phase III trial Same as a *randomised, double-blinded controlled trial*.

Pituitary gland The master *gland* of the body situated behind the nose and above the roof of the mouth. It controls the *thyroid gland*, the adrenal *gland*, the reproductive organs, growth and is important in lactation.

Placebo A psychologically beneficial effect of a medication or procedure that in reality has no healing effect.

Post hoc analysis A type of statistical analysis making comparisons between subgroups defined in retrospect.

Post-partum thyroiditis An *autoimmune* condition affecting about 10% of women within a year of giving birth. There can be a phase of *thyroid overactivity* followed by transient underactivity and then normal *thyroid* function, but other variations can also occur.

Predatory journal A profiteering type of journal with low-quality standards that fails to scrutinise the material submitted for publication.

Primary paper/evidence A paper or evidence based on studies that have not been published previously.

Prospective study A study that collects data as they become available.

Protein A large molecule made up of amino acids.

Radioiodine (or radioactive iodine) A form of iodine that is radioactive. It is used as a treatment for some types of *thyroid* overactivity. Very small doses of radioiodine are also sometimes used to scan the *thyroid*.

Randomised controlled clinical trial A type of study whereby different treatments are allocated to groups of patients at random.

Randomised, double-blinded controlled trial A type of study whereby different treatments are allocated to groups of patients at random and neither patient nor researcher knows which treatment corresponds to which patient until the study is complete.

Range A statistical term which is the difference between the smallest and largest measurement.

Receptor A chemical molecule made up primarily by proteins that binds a *hormone*. The fit is very specific and a receptor will generally only bind a particular *hormone*. Receptors are located either on the surface or the inside of cells. The binding of a *hormone* with a receptor is like a key and lock that is the first step in a series of reactions that leads to a response by a cell. So, binding of *TSH* with its receptor on the surface of *thyroid* cells makes the *thyroid* cell produce more *thyroid hormones*. The binding of *T3* to its receptor inside the cell makes that cell produce more energy.

Retrospective study A study that uses past records as the main information.

Sample size The number of participants in a study.

Sample size calculation A method for working out how many patients will be needed for a study.

Secondary paper/evidence A paper or evidence that discusses *primary papers/evidence*

Selection bias A limitation in a study whereby the subjects chosen differ consistently from the population of interest and skew the results in a particular direction.

Sinus tachycardia Rapid, regular heartbeat, more than 100 beats per minute. A common finding in people with an overactive *thyroid,* or when overtreated with *thyroid hormones.*

Standard deviation A statistical term that measures of the spread of the data around the average.

Statistical power The ability of a study design to give a clear answer.

Statistical significance A process that involves calculating whether one can be reasonably confident that if a study or experiment were to be repeated, the findings will be similar to what has been already observed.

Study oversight A process that is intended to ensure that research is conducted according to the rules of ethics and good practice.

Subacute thyroiditis Inflammation of the *thyroid* due to a viral infection. It is also called *De Quervain thyroiditis* or *viral thyroiditis.*

Subclinical hyperthyroidism *Thyroid* overactivity, which is so mild that it causes no symptoms and the diagnosis is made by blood tests. Typically, the serum *TSH* is less than the lower limit of normal with normal *FT3 and FT4.*

Subclinical hypothyroidism Also called 'compensated *hypothyroidism*' is a subtle type of *thyroid* underactivity, which is so mild that it causes no symptoms and the diagnosis is made by blood tests. It is defined as a serum *TSH* above the upper limit of normal but less than 10 mU/litre, associated with a normal *FT4* level.

Surrogate measure A convenient substitute to a harder outcome relevant to the question of what is clinically important.

Systematic review A type of publication that focuses on a specific topic or question and considers all the relevant evidence, but unlike *narrative reviews* it uses clearly defined methods for selecting the relevant evidence.

T3 One of the *hormones* that the *thyroid gland* makes. Also known as *liothyronine* and *L-T3*. The number 3 refers to the number of iodine atoms in the molecule. The letter 'L' indicates that the molecule is the left optic isomer. Optical isomers are structures of molecules that are mirror images of each other. Only the left isomer of T3 is biologically active. T3 is the principal active *thyroid hormone*.

T4 One of the *hormones* that the *thyroid* makes. Also known as *thyroxine, levothyroxine* and *L-T4*. The number 4 refers to the number of iodine atoms in the molecule. The letter 'L' indicates that the molecule is the left optic isomer. Optical isomers are structures of molecules that are mirror images of each other. Only the left isomer of T4 is biologically active. T4 is converted into *T3* in many tissues by *deiodinase enzymes*. T4 has some direct effects on cells, but it is regarded largely as a 'pro-*hormone*' that has to be converted to *T3* to act on cells.

TFT Stands for thyroid function tests. The full panel of TFTs includes *FT3, FT4* and *TSH*.

Thyroid An *endocrine gland* situated in the neck that make *thyroid hormones*.

Thyroid cartilage Same as Adam's apple. A firm structure in the neck above the *thyroid gland*.

Thyroid hormones *Hormones* that are made in the *thyroid gland*. The two main *thyroid hormones* are *T3* and *T4*. The *thyroid gland* also makes another *hormone* called *calcitonin* which has totally different function to *T3 and T4* and is involved in regulation of calcium.

Thyroid peroxidase An *enzyme* found in the *thyroid gland* that is involved in the production of *thyroid hormones*.

Thyroid uptake scintigram A type of scan of the *thyroid gland* whereby a miniscule amount of radioactive tracer is given by injection and pictures are taken of the *thyroid gland*. This type of scan can help doctors work out the cause of an overactive *thyroid*.

Thyroidectomy An operation to remove part or all of the *thyroid gland*.

Thyroiditis Inflammation of the *thyroid gland*.

Thyroglobulin A large *protein* made in the *thyroid gland* and used to store *thyroid hormones*.

Thyroglobulin antibodies *Antibodies* made against *thyroglobulin*. They occur in *autoimmune thyroid disease* and can be measured in blood.

Thyroxine One of the *thyroid hormones*, also known as *T4*.

Thyrotoxic/thyrotoxicosis The presence of excess *thyroid hormones* in the body.

Thyrotrophin/Thyrotropin It is also called *TSH* and *thyrotropin*. It is a *hormone* that is made by the *pituitary gland*. It acts on the *thyroid gland* and it drives it to make *thyroid hormones*.

Total T3 A blood test measuring of the total amount of *tri-iodothyronine* (T3) per unit volume in a blood sample (as opposed to '*free T3*').

Total T4 A blood test measuring of the total amount of *thyroxine (T4)* per unit volume in a blood sample (as opposed to '*free T4*').

TPO Stands for thyroid peroxidase, an *enzyme* found in *thyroid* cells, involved in making *thyroid hormones*.

TPOAb Stands for thyroid peroxidase antibodies. *Antibodies* that are directed to thyroid peroxidase. They are found in more than 90% of patients with *Hashimoto's thyroiditis* and in most patients with *Graves' disease*.

TRAb Stands for *TSH receptor antibodies*, a blood test for the *antibodies* that cause *Graves' disease*.

Translational research Research that focuses on turning the knowledge from *basic research* into treatments.

Transporter *Proteins* located in cells that control the passage of chemicals in and out of cell membranes.

Trepanation The drilling of holes in the skull.

TRH Stands for thyrotropin releasing hormone, a *hormone* made by the *hypothalamus,* that controls the secretion of *TSH*.

Trial A type of study usually involves a testing an intervention (treatment, procedure or medical device).

Tri-iodothyronine One of the naturally occurring *thyroid hormones*, also known as *T3*. Tri-iodothyronine is made in the *thyroid gland*, but also generated from *T4* in organs like the liver, muscle, brain and kidney. It is the active *thyroid hormone*.

TSH Stands for thyroid stimulating hormone. It is also called *thyrotropin* and *thyrotrophin*. It is a *hormone* that is made by the *pituitary gland*. It acts on the *thyroid gland* and it drives it to make *thyroid hormones*.

TSI Thyroid stimulating immunoglobulin. A blood test for *antibodies* to the *TSH receptor* using a biological (rather than a binding) *assay*. It is a diagnostic test for *Graves' disease* and is thought to be more sensitive than *TRAb*.

Uncontrolled clinical trial A type of study that lacks a comparative or 'control' group.

Validation A process that tests whether a measurement is reliable.

Viral thyroiditis Inflammation of the *thyroid* due to a viral infection. It is also known as *De Quervain thyroiditis* or *subacute thyroiditis*.

Index